LEARN TO READ CHINESE

An Introduction to the Language and Concepts
of Current *Zhongyi* Literature

by

Paul U. Unschuld

Volume Two

Sentence Structures, Stroke Order List of Characters,
General Glossary

Paradigm Publications
Brookline, Massachusetts, 1994

Electronic Layout pp. 1 - 284
  by Bo und Christine Hu, Stefan Rummel

Calligraphy of Stroke Order List pp. 285 - 311
  Dan-Wei Zhu-Mittag

General Glossary pp. 313 - 427
  by Anton Lachner

Library of Congress Cataloging in Publication Data

Unschuld, Paul U. (Paul Ulrich), 1943-
    [Chinesisch lesen lernen. English]
    Learn to read Chinese: an introduction to the language and concepts of current
Zhongyi literature / by Paul U. Unschuld.
        p.   cm.
    Includes bibliographical references and index.
    ISBN 0-912111-46-1 (v. 1) : $ 30.00. - ISBN 0-912111-47-X (v. 2) : $ 30.00
    1. Chinese language-Readers-Medicine, Chinese. 2. Medicine, Chinese. I. Title.
PL1117.5.M43U4713 1994
495.1′86421′02461 -dc20
                                                                94-16448
                                                                CIP

Copyright © 1994 Paul U.Unschuld

Paradigm Publications 44 Linden Street Brookline, Massachusetts 02146
U.S.A.

Printed in the United States of America

LEARN TO READ CHINESE
Volume Two

CONTENTS

Sentence Structures

LESSON 1: THE YINYANG DOCTRINE

Text 1.1

Sentence structures

Basic statement

中　医　用　　阴阳　学说
zhōng yī yòng yīnyáng xuéshuō

Chinese medicine employs the yinyang doctrine

why?

来 说明　基本 问题
lái shuōmíng jīběn wèntí

to explain basic issues

which
basic issues?

医学　　上的
yīxué shàngde

those **being present in** medicine

1. Adjunct statement

从而　成为　　思想 体系
cóng'ér chéngwéi sīxiǎng tǐxì

hence it constitutes a thought system

which
thought system?

中　医　　理论 的
zhōng yī lǐlùn de

(that) **of** Chinese medical theory

2. Adjunct statement

它 贯串　各个 方面
tā guànchuàn gège fāngmiàn

it permeates all aspects

1

which aspects?	在 zài		中 zhōng	医学 yīxué	中的 zhōngde

(those) **being present in** Chinese medicine

which are they?	生理, shēnglǐ,	病理, ... bìnglǐ, ...	治疗 zhìliáo	和 hé	药物 yàowù	等 děng

physiology, pathology, ... therapy and drugs

3. Adjunct statement

构成了 **gòuchéngle**	一 yī	整套 zhěngtào	医疗 yīliáo	方法 fāngfǎ

it **has generated** a complete therapy method

of what kind?	合乎 ... 的 héhū ... de

(one) conforming

conforming to what?	客观 kèguān	实际 shíjì

to objective reality

4. Adjunct statement

指导着 zhídǎozhe	临床 línchuáng	实践 shíjiàn

it guides the clinical practice

what clinical practice?	中 zhōng	医 yī	的 **de**

(that) **of** Chinese medicine

how?	灵活地 línghuóde

adaptably

Text 1.2

Sentence structures

<u>First unit of meaning</u>

Basic statement

阴阳 学说 是 一种 思想 方法
yīnyáng xuéshuō shì yīzhǒng sīxiǎng fāngfǎ

the yinyang doctrine is a thought method

what kind of a
thought method?

归纳出来(的)
guīnáchūlaí(de)

a.)

a conceptualized (one)

conceptualized
by whom?

古人
gǔrén

by the ancients

when?

在 观察 自然 现象 中
zài guānchá zìrán xiànxiàng zhōng

in observing natural phenomena

用 ... 的
yòng ... de

b.)

(one) being used

what for?

以 解释
yǐ jiěshì

to explain (something)

what?

自然 现象
zìrán xiànxiàng

these natural phenomena

Second unit of meaning

Basic statement

前　人　　发现
qián　rén　fāxiàn

earlier people discovered (something)

what?

万　物　　万　象　　　有　属性
wàn wù　　wàn xiàng　　yǒu shǔxìng

all　things, all　phenomena have attributes

how many?

两　种
liǎng zhǒng

two　kinds

which are they?

正　　　反
zhèng　　fǎn

(those) of norm and opposite

1. Adjunct statement

这种　　属性　是 对立　　而 又 统一的
zhèzhǒng shǔxìng　shì duìlì　　ér　yòu tǒngyīde

these　　attributes are antagonistic and yet unified

2. Adjunct statement

(这种　　属性)　存在 于 一切 事物 中
(zhèzhǒng shǔxìng)　cúnzài **yú** yīqiè　shìwù **zhōng**

(these　　attributes) exist **in** all　things

3. Adjunct statement

(前　人)　创立了　　阴阳 学说
(qián　rén)　chuànglìle　　yīnyáng xuéshuō

(earlier people) established the yinyang doctrine

4

4. Adjunct statement

| 用 这个 名词 |
| yòng zhège míngcí |

they used these terms

which terms?

| 阴 阳 |
| yīn yáng |

yin and yang

what for?

| 来 代表 关系 |
| lái dàibiǎo guānxì |

to represent relationships

which relationships?

| 所 存在着的 |
| **suǒ** cúnzàizhede |

a.)   **those which** are existing

where do they exist?

| 一切 事物 中 |
| yīqiè shìwù **zhōng** |

in all things

| 对立 统一 的 |
| duìlì tǒngyī **de** |

b.)   (those) **of** antagonism and unity

Third unit of meaning

Basic statement

| 如 天 为 阳, 地 为 阴 |
| rú tiān wéi yáng, dì wéi yīn |

e.g.: heaven is yang, earth is yin

1. - 3. Adjunct statement: structure identical with Basic statement

4. Adjunct statement

并　　　用 道理
bìng　　yòng dàolǐ

in addition they used principles

which principles?

相反　　　相成　　（的）
xiāngfǎn　　xiāngchéng **(de)**

a.)　　　　(that) **of** opposition and complementarity

对立　　　统一 的
duìlì　　　tǒngyī **de**

b.)　　　　(that) **of** antagonism and unity

why?

去 解释　变化
qù jiěshì　biànhuà

to　interpret changes

which
changes?

一切 事物 的
yíqiè　shìwù **de**

(those) **of** all　　things

where?

宇宙　间
yǔzhòu **jiān**

in the universe

Text 1.3

Sentence structures

<u>First unit of meaning</u>

Statement

中　医　　认为
zhōng　yī　　rènwéi

Chinese medicine　holds　　(something)

what does
it hold?

能　加以　　　　　解释
néng　jiāyǐ　　　　　jiěshì

(we) can　**provide** (something) **with** an explanation

what?

生理
shēnglǐ

physiology

what
physiology?

人　体　的
rén　tǐ　**de**

(that) **of** the human body

how can it
be explained?

用　　阴阳 学说 来
yòng　yīnyáng xuéshuō **lái**

with the yinyang doctrine

<u>Second unit of meaning</u>

Basic statement

性质　属　于 动
xìngzhì　shǔ　yú dòng

the nature　is associated with movement

what nature?

阳 的
yáng **de**

(that) of yang

1. Adjunct statement: structure identical with Basic statement

2. Adjunct statement

阳 有 能力
yáng yǒu nénglì

yang has an ability

which
ability?

保卫 的
bǎowèi **de**

(one) of safeguarding

what does
it safeguard?

体 表
tǐ biǎo

the body's exterior

3. Adjunct statement: structure identical with 2. Adjunct statement

<u>Third unit of meaning</u>

Basic statement

代表 皮 毛 ... 等
dàibiǎo pí máo ... děng

it represents skin and hair ...

whose skin
and hair ...?

体 表
tǐ biǎo

(those) of the body's exterior

by what?

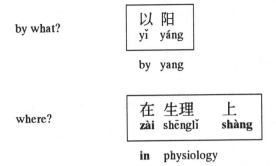

以	阳
yǐ	yáng

by yang

where?

在	生理	上
zài	shēnglǐ	**shàng**

in physiology

1. Adjunct statement: structure identical with Basic statement

2. Adjunct statement

并	以 ...	为 阴
bìng	yǐ ...	wéi yīn

in addition it considers ... as yin

what does it
consider as yin?

五	脏	主	藏
wǔ	zàng	zhǔ	cáng

the five depots master storage

what do they store?

精	气
jīng	qì

the essential qi

3. Adjunct statement: structure identical with 2. Adjunct statement

<u>Fourth unit of meaning</u>

Basic statement

(中	医)	分
(zhōng	yī)	fēn

(Chinese medicine) differentiates

9

on the basis of what?	从　　位置　上 **cóng**　wèizhì　**shàng**

on the basis of locations

that is?	上　焦　为　阳, ... shàng jiāo　wći yáng, ...

the upper burner is　yang, ...

Fifth unit of meaning: structure identical with Fourth unit of meaning

Sixth unit of meaning

Basic statement	(中　医)　用 (zhōng　yī)　yòng

(Chinese medicine) uses　(something)

what?	属性 shǔxìng

the nature

what nature?	阴　阳　的 yīn　yáng　de

(that) **of** yin or yang

which are they?	存在着 **cúnzàizhe**

(those) **being inherent**

where?	每一　处　都 **měiyī** chù　**dōu**

in **each**　locality

10

why?

以　说明
yǐ　shuōmíng

to　elucidate

to elucidate what?

特有的　　性质　和 特殊的功能
tèyǒude　　xìngzhì　hé　tèshūde　gōngnéng

characteristic qualities and specific　functions

which qualities
and functions?

生理　　的
shēnglǐ　　de

(those) of physiology

Text 1.4

Sentence structures

First unit of meaning

Basic statement

(中 医)	区别
(zhōng yī)	qūbié

(Chinese medicine) distinguishes (something)

on what basis?

根据	部位	和	性质
gēnjù	bùwèi	hé	xìngzhì

on the basis   of location and nature

what location and
nature?

发	病	的
fā	bìng	de

(that) **of** a developing illness

what does it
distinguish?

表	症	属	阳
biǎo	zhèng	shǔ	yáng

    a.)   the exterior pathoconditions belong to the yang

    b. - d.: structure identical with a.

Second unit of meaning

Basic statement

机能	衰弱	多	为	不足
jīnéng	shuāiruò	duō	wéi	bùzú

functional weaknesses often are   insufficiencies

insufficiencies of
what?

阳	的
yáng	de

of yang

for example?

如 少　　　气, 懒 言, ... 等
rú　shǎo　　qì,　lǎn　yán, ...　děng

e.g., diminished qi,　slow speech, ...

Adjunct statement: structure identical with Basic statement

Third unit of meaning

Statement

因而　　分　　　　作 四个 类型
yīnér　　fēn　　　zuò sìge　lèixíng

hence　it categorizes (them) into four　types

what is categorized
into four types?

一般　　症 状
yìbān　　zhèng zhuàng

the common patho- manifestations

namely?

阳 虚,　　阴 虚,　　阳 盛,　　阴 盛
yáng xū,　yīn xū,　yáng shèng,　yīn shèng

yang depletion, yin depletion, yang abundance, yin abundance

Fourth unit of meaning

Statement

归　　　　　阳 症
guī　　　　yáng zhèng

it identifies (something) as yang pathoconditions

what?

一切　　　亢进　　　的, 兴奋 的... 都
yīqìe　　kàngjìn　　de,　xìngfèn de ... dōu

all　　(cases) <u>of</u> hyperfunction,　<u>of</u> excitement ...

Adjunct statement: structure identical with Basic statement

13

Fifth unit of meaning

Basic statement

推 而 至	于	外	科
tuī ér zhì	yú	wài	kē

with regard to the external specialty

1. Adjunct statement

阳 症	是 红,	肿,	发热
yáng zhèng	shì hóng,	zhǒng,	fārè

yang pathoconditions are reddening, swelling, fever

2. Adjunct statement: structure identical with 1. Adjunct statement

14

Text 1.5

Sentence structures

<u>First unit of meaning</u>

Basic statement

分有	六个 纲要
fēnyǒu	liùge gāngyào

(Chinese medicine) distinguishes six   **basic categories**

in what
regard?

如	以	脉	诊	来	说
rú	yǐ	mài	zhěn	lái	shuō

e.g., **in regard to** pulse diagnosis

1. Adjunct statement

分	迟	和	数
fēn	chí	hé	shuò

it distinguishes retarded and frequent (pulses)

in what
regard?

在	至	数	上
zài	zhì	shù	**shàng**

in regard to arrival frequency

2. and 3. Adjunct statement: structure identical with 1. Adjunct statement

<u>Second unit of meaning</u>

Basic statement

数,	浮,	滑	属	于 阳
shuò,	fú,	huá	shǔ	yú yáng

frequent, surface, smooth belong to   yang

1. Adjunct statement: structure identical with Basic statement

2. Adjunct statement

阴	脉	见	于	阴	症
yīn	mài	xiàn	yú	yīn	zhèng

yin pulses appear with yin pathoconditions

3. Adjunct statement: structure identical with 2. Adjunct statement

Third unit of meaning

Basic statement

变化	属	于	病	变
biànhuà	shǔ	yú	bìng	biàn

changes belong to   the pathological changes

which changes?

舌	质	的
shé	zhì	de

(those) **of** tongue substance

to which
pathological
changes?

血液	的
xuèyè	de

(to those) **of** blood

in what regard?

以	舌	诊	来	说
yǐ	shé	zhěn	**lái**	**shuō**

in regard to tongue diagnosis

1. Adjunct statement

色	见	红	绛
sè	xiàn	hóng	jiàng

the color appears red   or crimson

what does
that mean?

是	血	热	属	阳
shì	xuè	rè	shǔ	yáng

this is   blood heat; it belongs to the yang

16

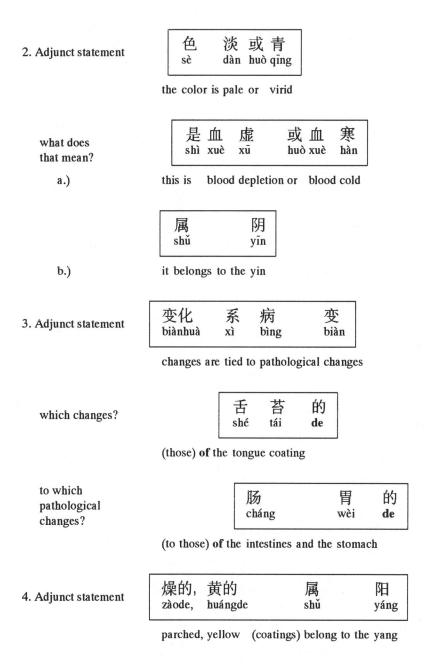

2. Adjunct statement

色　淡　或　青
sè　dàn　huò qīng

the color is pale or   virid

what does
that mean?

是 血 虚　或 血 寒
shì xuè xū　huò xuè hàn

a.)   this is   blood depletion or blood cold

属　　　阴
shǔ　　　yīn

b.)   it belongs to the yin

3. Adjunct statement

变化　系　病　　变
biànhuà　xì　bìng　　biàn

changes are tied to pathological changes

which changes?

舌　苔　的
shé　tái　de

(those) **of** the tongue coating

to which
pathological
changes?

肠　　　胃　的
cháng　　wèi　de

(to those) **of** the intestines and the stomach

4. Adjunct statement

燥的，黄的　　属　阳
zàode,　huángde　shǔ　yáng

parched, yellow   (coatings) belong to the yang

5. Adjunct statement: structure identical with 4. Adjunct statement

17

Text 1.6

Sentence structures

<u>First unit of meaning</u>

Basic statement

用	汗	法
yòng	hàn	fǎ

(Chinese medicine) applies sudorific patterns

when?

表	症
biǎo	zhèng

in cases of exterior pathoconditions

in what
regard?

在	治疗	上
zài	zhìliáo	shàng

in regard to therapy

1. - 3. Adjunct statement: structure identical with Basic statement

4. Adjunct statement

都	含有	意义
dōu	hányǒu	yìyì

all   have   a significance

which significance?

阴阳	的
yīnyáng	de

(one in terms) **of** the yinyang   (doctrine)

<u>Second unit of meaning</u>

Basic statement

主要	是
zhǔyào	shì

the important (thing) is

18

1. Adjunct statement

阳	胜		则		阴	病
yáng	shèng		zé		yīn	bìng

when yang dominates then the yin is ill

2. Adjunct statement: structure identical with 1. Adjunct statement

3. Adjunct statement

重	寒	现		热	象
chóng	hán	xiàn		rè	xiàng

doubled cold **brings forth** heat signs

4. Adjunct statement: structure identical with 3. Adjunct statement

Text 1.7

Sentence structures

<u>First unit of meaning</u>

Statement

分别	气	味
fēnbié	qì	wèi

(Chinese medicine) distinguishes qi   and flavor

in which
regard?

药	性
yào	xìng

(in regard to) drug qualities

which drug
qualities?

中	药	的
zhōng	yào	**de**

(those) **of** Chinese drugs

<u>Second unit of meaning</u>

Basic statement

一般	以	气	为 阳
yìbān	yǐ	qì	wéi yáng

generally, it considers qi to be   yang

Adjunct statement

味	为 阴
wèi	wéi yīn

(it considers) flavor to be   yin

<u>Third unit of meaning</u>

Basic statement

气	分	四	种
qì	fēn	sì	zhǒng

the qi   is distinguished into four types

20

1. Adjunct statement

寒	凉	属	阴
hán	liáng	shǔ	yīn

cold and cool belong to yin

2. Adjunct statement: structure identical with 1. Adjunct statement
3. Adjunct statement: structure identical with Basic statement
4. and 5. Adjunct statement: structure identical with 1. Adjunct statement

<u>Fourth unit of meaning</u>

Basic statement

称做	阳	药
chēngzuò	yáng	yào

(certain drugs) are called   yang drugs

which drugs?

具有 ...	的
jùyǒu ...	de

(those) possessing   (something)

what do they possess?

辛	热	性
xīn	rè	xìng

acrid and hot qualities

for example?

附子,	肉桂,	干姜	等
fūzǐ,	ròuguì,	gānjiāng	děng

fuzi,   rougui, ganjiang

1. Adjunct statement

能 升	能 散
néng shēng	néng sàn

they can   ascend and they can   disperse

2. Adjunct statement: structure identical with Basic statement
3. Adjunct statement: structure identical with 1. Adjunct statement

Fifth unit of meaning

Basic statement

也	叫	阳	药
yě	jiào	yáng	yào

they too are called yang drugs

which ones?

有	作用	的
yǒu	zuòyòng	**de**

(those) **having** a function

which function?

芳香	健	胃
fāngxiāng	jiàn	wèi

they are aromatic and strengthen the stomach

for example?

如 砂仁,	豆蔻 等
rú shārén,	dòukòu děng

e.g. sharen and doukou

Adjunct statement: structure identical with Basic statement

22

Text 1.8

Sentence structures

<u>First unit of meaning</u>

Basic statement

阴　　阳　是 概括性　代名词
yīn　　yáng shì gàikùoxìng dàimíngcí

yin and yang are general　　synonyms

of what
meaning?

对立　　　统一　的
duìlì　　　tǒngyì　de

(with the meaning) **of** antagonism and unity

which antagonism
and unity?

事物
shìwù

(those of all) things

Adjunct statement

(阴阳)　　可以 包括
(yīnyáng)　kěyǐ　bāokùo

(yin and yang) can　　include (something)

what is it?

对立,　都
duìlì,　**dōu**

all antagonisms

which antagonism?

不论　　　　　物质 的,
búlùn　　　　　wùzhì **de**,

<u>regardless of whether</u> those **of** matter,

机能　的　　部位　的
jīnéng　**de**　　bùwèi　**de**

of function,　or **of** position　<u>are concerned</u>

23

Second unit of meaning

Basic statement

应该　　　明确
yīnggāi　　míngquè

it should be made clear

what should
be made clear?

中　医　应用
zhōng yī　yìngyòng

Chinese medicine applies　(something)

what does
it apply?

阴阳
yīnyáng

the yinyang (doctrine)

how?

广泛地
guǎngfànde

extensively

to what?

于 各个 方面
yú gège　fāngmiàn

to all　realms

1. Adjunct statement

都 是 所　　指的
dōu shì suǒ　　zhǐde

all are **those which** are referring to (something)

what do they
refer to?

实有
shíyǒu

facts

2. Adjunct Statement

要	理解	道理
yào	lǐjiě	dàolǐ

if someone wishes to understand the principles

which principles?

运用	阴阳 的
yùnyòng	yīnyáng **de**

(those) **of** applying the yinyang (doctrine)

by whom?

中	医
zhōng	yī

by Chinese medicine

then what?

必须	通过	临症
bìxū	tōngguò	línzhèng

it is essential to pass through clinical (experience)

3. Adjunct statement

能	明白	实际	作用
néng	míngbái	shíjì	zuòyòng

it is possible to understand the practical applications

which practical applications?

所	起的
suǒ	<u>qǐde</u>

those which are <u>being brought forth</u>

by what?

阴阳
yīnyáng

by the yinyang (doctrine)

when?

只	有	通过	临症
zhǐ	**yǒu**	tōngguò	línzhèng

only **after having** passed through clinical (experience)

Third unit of meaning

Basic statement

例如 热 属 于 阳
lìrú rè shǔ yú yáng

e.g., heat belongs to yang

1. Adjunct statement

但 热 有 不 同
dàn rè yǒu bù tóng

but heat has dis- similarities

namely?

表 里,
biǎo lǐ,

a.) (those of) exterior or interior (heat),

虚 实 的
xū shí de

b.) (those) **of** depletion and **of** repletion

2. Adjunct statement

当 用 汗 法
dāng yòng hàn fǎ

it is appropriate to use a sudorific pattern

when?

发热
fārè

(in case of) fever

which fever?

引起的
yǐnqǐde

(one) **being set off**

set off by what?

伤　　　　风
shāng　　　fēng

a.) by harm caused by wind

感冒
gǎnmào

b.) by a **common cold**

3. Adjunct statement

叫做 疏散　　　解　　　表
jiàozuò shūsàn　　jiě　　biǎo

this is called　dispersion and opening the exterior

4. and 6. Adjunct statement: structure identical with 2. Adjunct statement
5. and 7. Adjunct statement: structure identical with 3. Adjunct statement

Fourth unit of meaning

Basic statement

热 属　于 阳
rè　shǔ　yú yáng

heat belongs to　yang

1. Adjunct statement

这 是　一般 情况
zhè shì　yìbān qíngkuàng

this is　a general condition

2. Adjunct statement

属　　于　　表　　是 机动的
shǔ　　yú　　biǎo　　shì jīdòngde

the association with the exterior, ... is　a flexible　(adaptation)

what association?

热 的
rè　de

(that) **of** heat

27

LESSON 2: THE FIVE PHASES DOCTRINE

Text 2.1

Sentence structures

<u>First unit of meaning</u>

Statement

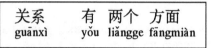

the five phases are wood, fire, soil, ...

<u>Second unit of meaning</u>

Basic statement

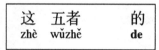

the relationships have two aspects

which relationships?

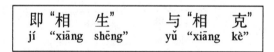

(those) **of** these five (phases)

Adjunct statement

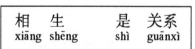

these are "mutual engendering" and "mutual restraint"

<u>Third unit of meaning</u>

Statement

相 生	是	关系
xiāng shēng	shì	guānxì

mutual engendering is a relationship

of what kind?

> 相互　资生　和　助长　的
> xiānghù zīshēng hé zhúzhǎng **de**

(one) **of** mutual   creation and support

Fourth unit of meaning

Basic statement

> 相　　生　　关系　　是　这样　的
> xiāng　shēng　guānxì　shì　zhè yàng **de**

the "mutual engendering" relationships are **of** this kind:

which relationships?

> 五　行　中的
> wǔ　xíng　**zhōngde**

(those) **being among** the five phases

1. Adjunct statement

> 木　生　　火
> mù　shēng　huǒ

wood generates fire

2. - 5. Adjunct statement: structure identical with 1. Adjunct statement

Fifth unit of meaning

Basic statement

> 可以 看出
> kěyǐ　kànchū

(we) can   see   (something)

from where?

> 从　　　关系　　中
> cóng　　guānxì　**zhōng**

from **within** the relationships

from which
relationships?

相　　生　　　　的
xiāng　shēng　　　de

(from those) **of** mutual engendering

what mutual
engendering?

五　行
wǔ　xíng

(that) of the five phases

what can
we see?

任何一　行　有　　两个　方面
rènhéyī　xíng　yǒu　liǎngge　fāngmiàn

each　　phase has　　two　　aspects

which aspects?

生　　　我和我生
shēng　　wǒ hé wǒ shēng

literally:

(another one) generates me and I generate (another one)

1. Adjunct statement

以　木　为　　例
yǐ　mù　wéi　lì

take wood as　an example

2. Adjunct statement

生　　　我者 为 水
shēng　　wǒ **zhě** wéi shuǐ

what generates me　　is　water

3. Adjunct statement

我 生者　为 火
wǒ　shēngzhě wéi huǒ

what I　generate is　fire

4. Adjunct statement

借　　母　子 关系　来 说
jiè　　mǔ　zǐ guānxì　lái shuō

take the mother son relationship to　explain (this)

30

5. Adjunct statement

水 为 母
shuǐ wéi mǔ

water is the mother

whose mother?

木 之
mù zhī

(that) **of** wood

6. Adjunct statement: structure identical with 5. Adjunct statement

Sixth unit of meaning

Statement

类推
lèituī

(we) deduce analogously

what?

其它 四 行
qítā sì xíng

the other four phases

analogously with what?

以 此
yǐ cǐ

(analogously) with this (example)

Text 2.2

Sentence structures

Statement

相	克	是	关系
xiāng	kè	shì	guānxì

mutual restraint is   a relationship

of what kind?

相互	约制	和	克服	的
xiānghù	yuēzhì	hé	kèfú	**de**

(one) **of** mutual   restrictions and overcoming

Second unit of meaning

Basic statement

相	克	关系	是
xiāng	kè	guānxì	shì

the " mutual restraint" relationship is (as follows):

which relationship?

五	行	中的
wǔ	xíng	**zhōngde**

(that) **being among** the five phases

1. Adjunct statement

金	克	木
jīn	kè	mù

metal restrains wood

2. - 5. Adjunct statement: structure identical with 1. Adjunct statement

32

Third unit of meaning

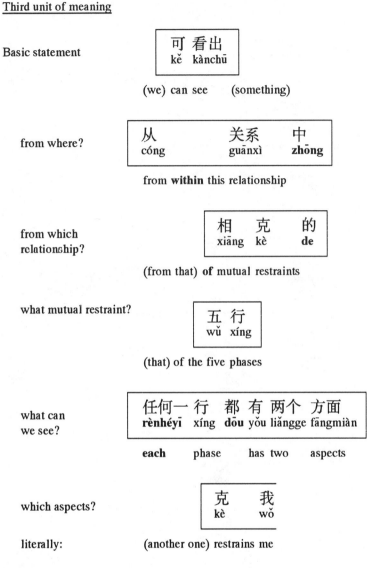

Basic statement

可 看出
kě kànchū

(we) can see   (something)

from where?

从   关系   中
cóng   guānxì   zhōng

from **within** this relationship

from which
relationship?

相   克   的
xiāng kè   **de**

(from that) **of** mutual restraints

what mutual restraint?

五 行
wǔ xíng

(that) of the five phases

what can
we see?

任何一 行   都 有 两个 方面
rènhéyī xíng **dōu** yǒu liǎngge fāngmiàn

each   phase   has two   aspects

which aspects?

克   我
kè   wǒ

literally:

(another one) restrains me

和 我 克
hé wǒ kè

and I   restrain (another one)

33

1. Adjunct statement

再 以 木 为 例
zài yǐ mù wéi lì

again, take wood as example

2. Adjunct statement

克 我者 为 金
kè wǒ zhě wéi jīn

what restrains me is metal

3. Adjunct statement

我 克者 为 土
wǒ kèzhě wéi tǔ

what I restrain is soil

4. Adjunct statement

金 为 所 不 胜者
jīn wéi **suǒ** bù shèngzhě

metal is **that which** (it) does not win against

what does not win
against the metal?

木
mù

the wood

5. Adjunct statement

土 为 所 胜者
tǔ wéi **suǒ** shèngzhě

soil is **that which** (it) wins against

what does win against
the soil?

木
mù

the wood

Text 2.3

Sentence structures

<u>First unit of meaning</u>

Basic statement

关系	不 是 (关系)
guānxì	bú shì (guānxì)

the relationships **are** not   (relationships)

which relationships?

它们 之间的
tāmen zhījiānde

(those) **among** them

among what?

上 述	两个 方面
shàng shù	liǎngge fāngmiàn

(among) the above mentioned two   aspects

which aspects?

相 生	和 相 克
xiāng shēng	hé xiāng kè

(those) of mutual engendering and mutual restraint

which engendering/
restraint?

五 行
wǔ xíng

(that) of the five phases

what kind of
relationships
are they not?

并 行 不 悖	(的)
bìng xíng bù beì	(de)

(those) **of** parallel moving, not touching

1. Adjunct statement

是	相互 为用 的
shì	xiānghù wéiyòng de

they are (those) **of** mutual usefulness

2. Adjunct statement

生　　　克　　之间　有　关系
shēng　　kè　　**zhījiān** yǒu guānxì

among engendering and restraint　　exist relationships

of what kind?

密切的
mìqiède

close (ones)

3. Adjunct statement

生　　　中　有　克
shēng　　**zhōng** yǒu kè

within engendering　　exists restraint

4. Adjunct statement: structure identical with 3. Adjunct statement

<u>Second unit of meaning</u>

Basic statement

这种　关系　　称做
zhèzhǒng guānxì　**chēngzuò**

this　　relationship **is called**

制　　　化　　　关系
zhì　　　huà　　　guānxì

"construction/counterreaction" relationship

which relationship?

相互　为用　　的
xiānghù wéiyòng **de**

(that) **of** mutual usefulness

1. Adjunct statement

木　克　　土
mù　kè　　tǔ

wood restrains soil

36

2. - 3. Adjunct statement: structure identical with 1. Adjunct statement

<u>Third unit of meaning</u>

Basic statement

制	化	关系
zhì	huà	guānxì

the construction/counterreaction relationship

是	必要	条件
shì	bìyào	tiáojiàn

is   an essential condition

of what?

维持	平衡 的
wéichí	pínghéng **de**

of maintaining a balance

1. Adjunct statement

否则	有	生	无 克
fǒuzé	**yǒu**	shēng	wú kè

otherwise **there is** engendering but no   restraint

2. Adjunct statement

必	使
bì	shǐ

this must cause (the following)

what?

盛者	更	盛
shèngzhě	**gèng**	shèng

the abundant to become **even more** abundant

3. Adjunct statement: structure identical with 1. Adjunct statement

Text 2.4

Sentence structures

<u>First unit of meaning</u>

Basic statement

还 有　　　反常　现象
hái **yǒu**　　　fǎncháng xiànxiàng

there is yet　　another unusual　phenomenon

where?

在　生　　　克　中
zài　shēng　　　kè　**zhōng**

within engendering and restraint

1. Adjunct statement

我　克者　克　　我
wǒ　**kèzhě**　kè　　wǒ

literally:

that what I　restrain restrains me

when?

有时
yǒushí

sometimes

how?

反来
fǎnlái

contrary (to what is normal)

2. Adjunct statement

克　　我者 为　　我 克
kè　　wǒ **zhě** wéi　　wǒ kè

literally:

what restrains me　is　what I　restrain

38

Second unit of meaning

Basic statement

水　克　火
shuǐ　kè　huǒ

water restrains fire

1. Adjunct statement

火 能 反过来 克　水
huǒ néng fǎnguòlái kè　shuǐ

fire can, conversely, restrain water

when?

在　某种　情况　下
zài　móuzhǒng qíngkuàng **xià**

under certain conditions

2. Adjunct statement

这 称做　"相　侮"
zhè **chēngzuò** "xiāng　wǔ"

that **is called** "mutual humiliation"

Third unit of meaning

Basic statement

凡是 均　　　有 一个 条件
fánshì jūn　　　yǒu yīgè tiáojiàn

all (relationships) have a precondition

which relationships?

相　生,　　相 克, ...
xiāng shēng,　　xiāng kè, ...

(those of) mutual engendering, mutual restraint, ...

1. Adjunct statement

气 充实
qì chōngshí

when the qi abounds

39

whose qi?

本身 之
běnshēn **zhǐ**

(that) **of** (a specific phase) itself

what will happen?

则 相 生
zé xiāng shēng

then there is mutual engendering

2. Adjunct statement

否则 不能 生
fǒu zé bù néng shēng

if not then it is not able to generate

3. Adjunct statement

气 有 余
qì yǒu yú

the qi (of a specific phase) has a surplus

what will happen?

则 能克 和侮
zé néng kè hé wǔ

then it can restrain and humiliate

restrain what?

所 胜
suǒ shèng

that (phase) **which** it (usually) wins against

and humiliate what?

所 不胜
suǒ bú shèng

that (phase) **which** it (usually) does not win against

3. Adjunct statement

（气） 不及
(qì) bù jí

(the qi) is not sufficient

what will happen?

则	不能	克	所		胜
zé	bù néng	kè	suǒ		shèng

then it is not able to restrain **that which** it (usually) wins against

and?

反	为乘	侮
fǎn	wéi chéng	wǔ

in contrast, it is   seized and humiliated

by what?

所		不 胜
suǒ		bù shèng

by **that which** (usually) does not win against it

Text 2.5

Sentence structures

<u>First unit of meaning</u>

Basic statement

运用	是	归纳起来
yùnyòng	shì	guīnàqilai

the application is   to conceptualize (something)

the application
of what?

五	行	在	中	医学	上	的
wǔ	xíng	**zài**	zhōng	yīxué	**shàng**	<u>de</u>

(that) <u>of</u> the five phases **in** Chinese medicine

to conceptualize
what?

自然	界	和	人体	组织
zìrán	jiè	hé	réntǐ	zǔzhī

the natural world and the human organism

how?

按	属性
àn	shǔxìng

a.)   **in accordance with** the characteristics

which characteristics?

五	行	的
wǔ	xíng	**de**

(those) **of** the five phases

在	一定的 情况	下
zài	yīdìngde qíngkuàng	**xià**

b.)   **under** specific   conditions

42

Adjunct statement

说明
shuōmíng

(we) explain   (something)

what?

相互 关系
xiānghù guānxì

the mutual relationships

which
relationships?

脏腑 之间的
zàngfǔ **zhījiānde**

(those) **being among** the organs

how are they
explained?

以   关系
yǐ   guānxì

by means of relationships

which
relationships?

生   克   的
shēng   kè   **de**

(those) **of** engendering and restraint

Second unit of meaning

Statement

可 从属
kě cóngshǔ

(we) can categorize (something)

what?

东， 南， 中， 西，   北
dōng, nán, zhōng, xī,   běi

a.)

east, south, center, west, and north

43

as what?

方位 的
fāngwèi de

(as dimensions) **of** the cardinal points

b. - f.: structure identical with a.

how?

依　　　　　　次序　来
yī　　　　　　cìxù　lái

in accordance with the sequence

which sequence?

木,　火,　土,　金,　　水　的
mù,　huǒ, tǔ,　jīn,　　shuǐ de

(that) **of** wood, fire, soil, metal, and water

in what regard?

自然 界　来说
zìrán jiè　lái shuō

in regard to the natural world

Text 2.6

Sentence structures

<u>First unit of meaning</u>

Basic statement

(中 医)	以	肝 ...	为	中心
(zhōng yī)	yǐ	gān ...	wéi	zhōngxīn

(Chinese medicine) holds the liver ... to be the center

in what regard?

在	人	体	方面
zài	rén	tǐ	**fāngmiàn**

in regard to the human body

Adjunct statement

联系	(肝,	心, ...)	到
liánxì	(gān	xīn, ...)	dào

it links (the liver, the heart ...) to (something)

to what?

七	窍, ...
qī	qiào, ...

to the seven orifices, ...

which seven orifices?

目,	舌,	口, ...	的
mù,	shé,	kǒu, ...	**de**

(those) **of** the eyes, the tongue, the mouth, ...

<u>Second unit of meaning</u>

Statement

可	结合起来	加以	分析
kě	jiéhéqilai	jiāyǐ	fēnxī

(we) can link and analyze (something)

what?

把 它们
bǎ tāmen

them

how?

从 直接 或 间接的关系
cóng zhíjiē huò jiànjiēde guānxì

starting from direct or indirect relationships

when?

明白了 后
míngbáile hòu

a.)　　　after one has understood

what?

这一 归类　　方法
zhèyì guīlèi　　fāngfǎ

this classification method

当　　接触 到　事物 时
dāng jiēchù dào shìwù sshí

b.)　　　when (we) touch on an item

which item?

属的
shǔde

(one) being related

related to what?

于　某　一 行　性质
yú mǒu yī xíng xìngzhì

to a certain phase nature

why?

以便 理解
yǐbiàn lǐjiě

to understand (something)

what?

| 这一 事物 的性质 |
| zhèyī shìwù de xìngzhì |

this   item's   nature

Text 2.7

Sentence structures

<u>First unit of meaning</u>

Statement

> 同样　是 指导 ...的
> tóngyàng shì zhǐdǎo ... de

(both) alike　　are guiding

what is guiding?

> 五 行　学说 和　阴阳 学说 一样
> wǔ xíng　xuéshuō hé　yīnyáng xuéshuō yīyàng

the five phases doctrine and the yinyang doctrine alike

doctrines of what?

> 中　医　的
> zhōng yī **de**

(those) **of** Chinese medicine

what do they guide?

> 临床　工作
> línchuáng gōngzuò

the clinical　work

what clinical work?

> 中　医　的
> zhōng yī **de**

(that) **of** Chinese medicine

<u>Second unit of meaning</u>

Basic statement

> **举例来说,** 如 木 性　条畅
> **jǔlìláishuō, rú** mù xìng tiáochàng

for example,　　wood nature is to pass freely

48

1. Adjunct statement

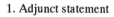

肝　气　应　　　舒畅
gān　qì　yīng　　shūchàng

the liver qi　should be unimpeded

2. Adjunct statement

郁
yù

when it is impeded

what will happen?

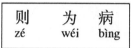

则　　　为　　病
zé　　　wéi　　bìng

then this is　an illness

3. Adjunct statement

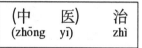

(中　　医)　　治
(zhōng　yī)　　zhì

(Chinese medicine) treats (such a condition)

how?

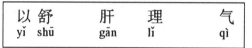

以 舒　　　肝　　理　　　　气
yǐ shū　　　gān　　lǐ　　　　qì

by　opening the liver and regulating the qi

Third unit of meaning

Basic statement

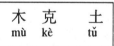

木　克　　土
mù　kè　　tǔ

wood restrains soil

1. Adjunct statement

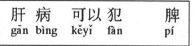

肝 病　可以 犯　　　脾
gān bìng　kěyǐ fàn　　pí

liver illness can　invade the spleen

49

2. Adjunct statement

应当	预为	防治
yīngdāng	yùwéi	fángzhì

it is appropriate to prepare a prevention

when?

未	犯		前
wèi	fàn		**qián**

before an invasion has occurred

3. Adjunct statement

已	发现	脾	病	时
yǐ	fāxiàn	pí	bìng	**shí**

when (a therapist) has already discovered a spleen illness

what happens then?

则	宜	疏	肝	健	脾
zé	yí	shū	gān	jiàn	pí

then it is advisable to dredge the liver and to strengthen the spleen

Fourth unit of meaning

Basic statement

水	能	生	木
shuǐ	néng	shēng	mù

water can engender wood

1. Adjunct statement

可	用	方法
kě	yòng	fāngfǎ

(we) can employ a method

which one?

滋 … 的
zī … de

an enriching (one)

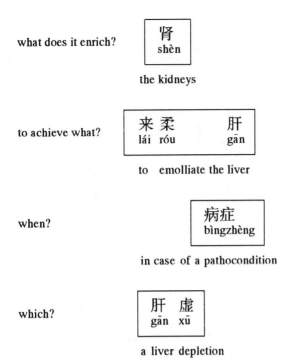

what does it enrich?

肾
shèn

the kidneys

to achieve what?

来 柔　　肝
lái róu　　gān

to　emolliate the liver

when?

病症
bìngzhèng

in case of a pathocondition

which?

肝　虚
gān　xū

a liver depletion

2. Adjunct statement: structure identical with Basic statement

3. Adjunct statement: structure identical with 1. Adjunct statement

Text 2.8

Sentence structures

<u>First unit of meaning</u>

Statement

其它	脏	病		是 处理的
qítā	zāng	bìng		shì chǔlǐde

other depot illnesses are dealt with

how?

按照	道理
ànzhào	dàolǐ

according to the principles

which principles?

相	生		相	克	的
xiāng	shēng		xiāng	kè	**de**

(those) **of** mutual engendering/mutual restraint

what engendering/
restraint?

五	行
wǔ	xíng

(that) of the five phases

for example?

用	培	土	生	金	法
yòng	péi	tǔ	shēng	jīn	fǎ

a.)

(we) use a "heap soil and generate metal" pattern

when?

肺	劳
fèi	láo

in case of lung taxation

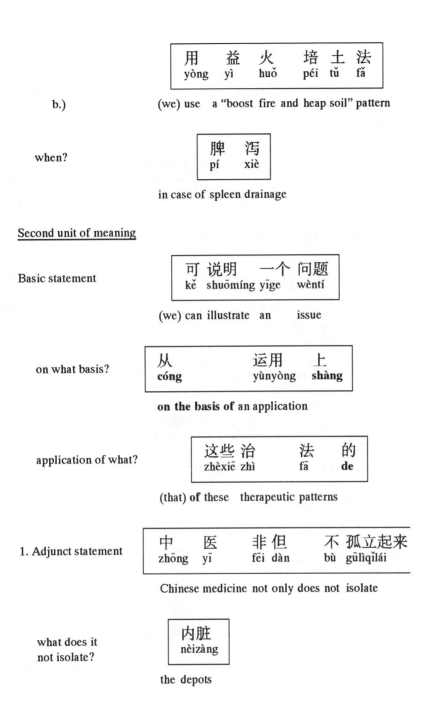

用	益	火	培	土	法
yòng	yì	huǒ	péi	tǔ	fǎ

b.)   (we) use   a "boost fire and heap soil" pattern

when?

脾	泻
pí	xiè

in case of spleen drainage

Second unit of meaning

Basic statement

可	说明	一个	问题
kě	shuōmíng	yīge	wèntí

(we) can illustrate   an   issue

on what basis?

从	运用	上
cóng	yùnyòng	**shàng**

on the basis of an application

application of what?

这些	治	法	的
zhèxiē	zhì	fǎ	**de**

(that) **of** these   therapeutic patterns

1. Adjunct statement

中	医	非	但	不	孤立起来
zhōng	yī	fēi	dàn	bù	gūlìqǐlái

Chinese medicine not only does not isolate

what does it
not isolate?

内脏
nèizàng

the depots

而且	重视	密切	联系
érqiě	zhòngshì	mìqiè	liánxì

but   it emphasizes close   relationships

which relationships?

内脏	之间的
nèizàng	zhījiānde

(those) **existing among** the depots

2. Adjunct statement

(中	医)	进行	治疗
(zhōng	yī)	jìnxíng	zhìliáo

(Chinese medicine) conducts a therapy

when?

在	甲	脏	有	病	时
zài	jiǎ	zàng	yǒu	bìng	**shí**

when a first depot has an illness

starting where?

从	乙	脏	或	丙	脏	来
cóng	yǐ	zàng	huò	bǐng	zàng	**lái**

from a second depot or   third depot

3. Adjunct statement

有	方法
yǒu	fāngfǎ

there exist patterns

which patterns?

"隔	一", ...
"gé	yī", ...

a.)   (the so-called) "separated by one (depot)", ...

和	虚	则 补 其 母, ...
hé	xū	zé bǔ qí mǔ, ...

b.)   and "when there is depletion, then fill its mother" ...

LESSON 3: THE CONDUITS AND NETWORK VESSELS

Text 3.1

Sentence structures

<u>First unit of meaning</u>

Statement

经	络	学说	是	组成	部分
jīng	luò	xuéshuō	shì	zǔchéng	bùfēn

the conduit/network doctrine is a constitutive element

what kind of an element?

重要的
zhòngyàode

an important (one)

where is it a constitutive element?

理论	体系	中
lǐlùn	tǐxì	**zhōng**

in the theoretical system

in which theoretical system?

中	医
zhōng	yī

(in that of) Chinese medicine

<u>Second unit of meaning</u>

Basic statement

它	为	一门	课程
tā	wéi	yīmén	kèchéng

it is one subject

what kind of a subject?

必	修的
bì	xiūde

(one that) must be studied

by whom?

医者
yīzhě

by physicians

1. Adjunct statement

贯穿　　各个 方面
guànchuān gège　fāngmiàn

it　penetrates all　　aspects

which aspects?

在 中　医　　的
zài zhōng　yī　　de

(those) **being** in　Chinese medicine

namely?

生理,　　病理　　诊断, ...
shēnglǐ,　bìnglǐ,　zhěnduàn, ...

physiology, pathology, diagnosis, ...

in which way?

和　　阴阳 五 行　学说　一样
hé　　yīnyáng wǔ xíng　xuéshuō yīyàng

with　the yinyang/five phases doctrines identical

2. Adjunct statement

并　　　　起有　重要的　作用
bìng　　　qǐyǒu　zhòngyàode zuòyòng

simultaneously it fulfills an important　function

Third unit of meaning

Basic statement

经　络　　　　网罗　　全 身
jīng　luò　　　wǎngluó　　quán shēn

the conduits/network (vessels) interconnect the entire body

1. Adjunct statement

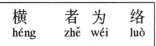

the straight ones are the conduits

2. Adjunct statement

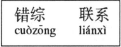

the crosswise ones are the network (vessels)

3. Adjunct statement

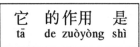

they form complicated relationships

<u>Fourth unit of meaning</u>

Statement

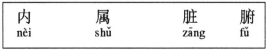

their   functions are (the following)

namely?

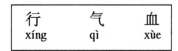

a.)   internally they connect with the depots and palaces

b.: structure identical with a.

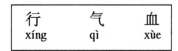

c.)   they transmit the qi and the blood

d. - f.: structure identical with c.

Statement

经	络		为	经	脉, ...
jīng	luò		wéi	jīng	mài, ...

the conduits/network (vessels) are the conduit vessels, ...

which conduits/
network(vessels)?

全	身
quán	shēn

(those) of the entire body

which conduits/
network(vessels)?

主要的
zhǔyàode

the important (ones)

58

Text 3.2

Sentence structures

<u>First unit of meaning</u>

Basic statement

分为　　　　　　阳　经　　阴　经
fēnwéi　　　　　yáng jīng　　yīn jīng

(we) divide (something) into yang conduits and yin conduits

into how many?

六　支
lìu　zhī

into six

what do we divide?

十二　经　脉
shí'èr　jīng　mài

the twelve conduit vessels

where?

其　　　　　　　　　　　中
qí　　　　　　　　　　　zhōng

among these (conduits and network vessels)

1. Adjunct statement

经　相　传
jīng　xiāng　chuán

the conduits mutually transmit (their contents)

how?

逐
zhú

successively

2. Adjunct statement

循行	脏 腑	头面, ...
xúnxíng	zāng fǔ	tóumiàn, ...

they permeate the depots/palaces, the head, ...

Second unit of meaning

Basic statement

经	别	是 别出
jīng	bié	shì biéchū

the conduit branches are offshoots

offshoots of what?

十二	经	脉	的
shí'èr	jīng	mài	**de**

of the twelve conduit vessels

1. Adjunct statement

构成	表	里	配合
gòuchéng	biǎo	lǐ	pèihé

they fashion the outside-inside combination

where?

在	阳 经	和	阴 经	之间
zài	yáng jīng	hé	yīn jīng	**zhījiān**

between the yang conduits and the yin conduits

2. Adjunct statement

着重	联系
zhuózhòng	liánxì

they emphasize connections

which connections?

于	深	部	的
yú	shēn	bù	**de**

(those) **existing** with deep-lying regions

3. Adjunct statement

经	筋	起	于	肢	末
jīng	jīn	qǐ	yú	zhī	mò

the conduit sinews arise from the limb ends

4. Adjunct statement

行	于	体	表
xíng	yú	tǐ	biǎo

they pass through the body's exterior

5. Adjunct statement: structure identical with 2. Adjunct statement

6. Adjunct statement

奇	经	八	脉	为 (脉)
qí	jīng	bā	mài	wéi (mài)

the **eight** extraordinary conduit   vessels are (vessels)

of what kind?

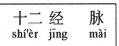

regulating (ones)

what do they regulate?

十二	经	脉
shí'èr	jīng	mài

the twelve conduit vessels

Text 3.3

Sentence structures

<u>First unit of meaning</u>

Basic statement

所以	经	脉	是	必由的	通路
suǒyǐ	jīng	mài	shì	bìyóude	tōnglù

hence the conduit vessels are essential pathways

essential for what?

气	血	运行
qì	xùe	yùnxíng

for qi and blood transmission

1. Adjunct statement

贯串	内	外,	上	下 …
guànchuán	nèi	wài,	shàng	xià, …

they penetrate   inner and outer, upper and lower, …

where?

在	人	体
zài	rén	tǐ

in the human body

2. Adjunct statement

从而	联系
cóng'ér	liánxì

hence   they connect (something)

what?

各	部分
gè	bùfēn

all   parts

of what?

人	体
rén	tǐ

of the human body

namely which?	包括	五 脏,		六 腑, …
	bāokuò	wǔ zāng,		lìu fǔ, …

this includes the five depots, the six palaces, ...

3. Adjunct statement	成为	有机的 统一	整体
	chéngwéi	yǒujīde tǒngyī	zhěngtǐ

they create   an organic   integrated whole

<u>Second unit of meaning</u>

Basic statement	由 阴		入 阳
	yóu yīn		rù yáng

from yin (regions) they enter yang (regions)

why?	由于	经 络		互相 衔接
	yóuyú	jīng luò		hùxiāng xiánjiē

because the conduits/network (vessels) are mutually linked

1. - 5. Adjunct statement: structure identical with Basic statement

6. Adjunct statement	气	血 流行
	qì	xuè líuxíng

the qi and the blood flow

7. Adjunct statement	循环 不	息
	xúnhuán bù	xī

they circulate without pause

8. Adjunct statement	所	谓	阴	阳	相	随
	suǒ	wèi	yīn	yáng	xiāng	**suí**

(that is) what is called "yin and yang **follow** each other"

9. Adjunct statement: structure identical with 8. Adjunct statement

10. Adjunct statement

(所	谓)	如	环 无	端
(suǒ	wèi)	rú	huán wú	duān

(that is what is called) "like a ring without end"

Text 3.4

Sentence structures

<u>First unit of meaning</u>

Basic statement

功能　以 ... 为 主
gōngnéng yǐ ...　wéi zhǔ

the functions **rest on ...**

which functions?

生理
shēnglǐ

the physiological (functions)

functions of what?

人　体
rén　tǐ

(those) of the human body

what do they rest on?

五　脏　　六　腑
wǔ zāng　lìu fǔ

the five depots and six palaces

Adjunct statement

经　络　　　　　起有 作用
jīng luò　　　　qǐyǒu zuòyòng

the conduits/network (vessels) play a role

what role?

重要的
zhòngyàode

an important (one)

65

in what regard?

使
shǐ

a.)   they cause (something)

what?

内	外	上	下	保持着	协调
nèi	wài	shàng	xià	bǎochízhe	xiétiáo

inner and outer, above and below maintain a harmony

which inner/outer,
above and below?

人　体
rén　tǐ

(those) of the human body

what kind of harmony?

平衡　的
pínghéng **de**

(one) **of** balance

进行　活动
jìnxíng　huódòng

b.)   they carry out activities

which activities?

有机的 整体
yǒujǐde　zhěngtǐ

(those) of an organic　whole

Second unit of meaning

Basic statement

经	络	学说	是	形成的
jīng	luò	xuéshuō	shì	xíngchéngde

the conduit/network doctrine was formed

when?	在　　长时期的　临症　实践　中
	zài　chángshíqíde línzhèng shíjiàn zhōng

during long-term　clinical　practice

by whom?	前　　人
	qián　rén

by former people

how?	根据　分析　研究
	gēnjù　fēnxī　yánjiū

based on analytical research

research of what?	治疗　效果　的
	zhìliáo xiàoguǒ de

of therapy results

which therapy results?	无数　　病　例
	wúshù　bìng lì

(those) of innumerable illness cases

Third unit of meaning

Basic statement	用　　经　　络
	yòng　jīng　luò

(we) employ the conduit/network (doctrine)

why?	来 分析　症　候
	lái fēnxī　zhèng hòu

to　analyze the illness signs

67

Adjunct statement

能 作
néng zuò

(we) can   consider (such an analysis)

as what?

为   准则 之 一
wéi   zhǔnzé zhī yī

as   **one** <u>of</u> the criteria

criteria of what?

辨	症	论	治	的
biàn	zhèng	lùn	zhì	**de**

of differentiating pathoconditions and **of** determining a therapy

Text 3.5

Sentence structures

<u>First unit of meaning</u>

Statement

传	变	由	表	入 里, ...
chuán	biàn	yóu	biǎo	rù lǐ, ...

transmissions/changes occur from outside to inside, ...

which transmissions/
changes?

外	邪	的
wài	xié	**de**

(those) **of** external evils

which external
evils?

一般
yībān

general (ones)

how do they occur?

大多	通过	经	络
dàduō	tōngguò	jīng	luò

mostly through the conduits and network (vessels)

<u>Second unit of meaning</u>

Basic statement

以	病	来	说
yǐ	bìng	lái	shuō

(we) take an illness to explain (this)

which illness?

真	中	风
zhēn	zhòng	fēng

being truly struck by wind

1. Adjunct statement

轻	者	中	络
qīng	zhě	zhòng	luò

minor ones hit   the network (vessels)

2. Adjunct statement

症		见	肌肤	麻木, ...
zhèng		xiàn	jīfū	mámù, ...

as pathoconditions appear skin   insensitivity, ...

3. and 4. Adjunct statement: structure identical with 2. Adjunct statement

<u>Third unit of meaning</u>

Basic statement

疾病	会	反映出来
jíbìng	huì	fǎnyìngchūlái

illnesses can appear

which illnesses?

发生的
fāshēngde

(those) having developed

from where?

自	内	脏
zì	nèi	zāng

from the inner depots

where can they
appear?

在	经	络
zài	jīng	luò

in the conduits and network (vessels)

in which?

所	属
suǒ	shǔ

in **those which** belong (to them)

70

1. Adjunct statement

如 肺, 心 有 邪
rú fèi, xīn yǒu xié

e.g., lung or heart have an evil

what happens?

其 气 留 于 两 肘
qí qì líu yú liǎng zhǒu

its qi settles in the two elbows

2. - 4. Adjunct statement: structure identical with 1. Adjunct statement

Fourth unit of meaning

Basic statement

气 留
qì líu

the qi settles

what happens?

则 痛
zé tòng

then pain (results)

Adjunct statement

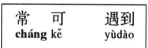
常 可 遇到
cháng kě yùdào

(we) can **often** encounter (that)

where?

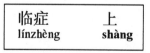
临症 上
línzhèng **shàng**

in clinical (reality)

71

Text 3.6

Sentence structures

<u>First unit of meaning</u>

Statement

经	络	是	依据	之 一
jīng	luò	shì	yījù	<u>zhī</u> yī

the conduits/network (vessels) are **one** <u>of</u> the foundations

one of which
foundations?

重要
zhòngyào

(one of) the important (foundations)

where?

在 临症 治疗 上
zài línzhèng zhìliáo **shàng**

in clinical therapy

<u>Second unit of meaning</u>

Basic statement

针刺 合谷 穴
zhēncì hégǔ xuè

(we) needle the hegu hole

where?

手 上
shǒu **shàng**

on the hand

with what effect?

能 治 龈 肿 ...
néng zhì yín zhǒng ...

this can treat gum swelling ...

what kind of needling
is that?

大家	熟悉的
dàjiā	shúxīde

one **being known** to everybody

1. Adjunct statement

刺	足 三里 穴
cì	zú sānlǐ xuè

(we) prick the leg sanli hole

with what effect?

能 治 胃 病
néng zhì wèi bìng

this can treat stomach ailments

2. Adjunct statement

这些 都 是 作用
zhèxiē dōu shì zuòyòng

these all are effects

which effects?

所	起的
suǒ	qǐde

those which have been stimulated

how?

通过	经	络
tōngguò	jīng	luò

through the conduits and network (vessels)

Third unit of meaning

Basic statement

经	络	有 关系
jīng	luò	yǒu guānxì

the conduits and network (vessels) have relationships

with what?	于 处 方　　用 药 yú chǔ fāng　　yòng yào

with writing prescriptions and using drugs

1. Adjunct statement	分属　　　　十二 经 fēnshǔ　　　shí'èr jīng

(we) assign (something) to the twelve conduits

what?	主 治　　功能 zhǔ zhì　　gōngnéng

the main therapeutic functions

which main functions?	药物 的 yàowù de

(those) **of** drugs

where?	中　药学　　上 zhōng yàoxué　shàng

in Chinese pharmaceutics

2. Adjunct statement	见　病 jiàn bìng

(we) observe an illness

what kind of illness?	那 一　　经 nà yī　　jīng

(one in) that particular conduit

what happens?	用 药 yòng yào

(we) use a drug

what kind of drug?

那	一	类
nà	yī	lèi

(one) of that particular type

Text 3.7

Sentence structures

<u>First unit of meaning</u>

Basic statement

麻黄 入　　太 阳 经
máhuáng rù　　tài　yáng jīng

mahuang enters the major yang conduit

1. and 2. Adjunct statement: structure identical with Basic statement

<u>Second unit of meaning</u>

Basic statement

三 药 能 治疗 头 痛
sān　yào　néng zhìliáo tóu tòng

three drugs can treat　headache

which drugs?

以上 均
yǐshàng jūn

(those mentioned) above　all alike

which headache?

风　　寒
fēng　　hán

(that caused by) wind　and cold

1. Adjunct statement

痛　　在 后脑 及　　项 者
tòng　zài hòunǎo jí　　xiàng **zhě**

when pain occurs in the afterbrain and in the nape

what is that?	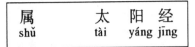

this belongs to the major yang conduit

what is to be done?	用 麻黄 yòng máhuáng

use   mahuang

2. and 3. Adjunct statement: structure identical with 1. Adjunct statement

<u>Third unit of meaning</u>

Basic statement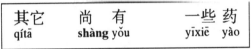

furthermore   there are **still** some drugs

1. Adjunct statement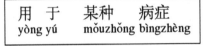

they are used against specific   illness-pathoconditions

when?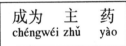

often

2. Adjunct statement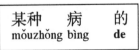

they represent master drugs

which master drugs?
```
某种    病    的
mǒuzhǒng bìng   de
```

those **of** specific   illnesses

3. Adjunct statement

辛夷	用	于	鼻	塞
xīnyí	yòng	yú	bí	sè

xinyi is used against nasal blockages

4. Adjunct statement: structure identical with 3. Adjunct statement

5. Adjunct statement

都	是	来的
dōu	shì	láide

all are (those) having come

from where?

从	分	经	上
cóng	fēn	jīng	shàng

via   different conduits

Text 3.8

Sentence structures

<u>First unit of meaning</u>

Basic statement

一般	认为
yībān	rènwéi

generally (people) assume (something)

what?

经	络	学说	指导	理论	跟据
jīng	luò	xuéshuǒ	zhǐdaǒ	lǐlùn	gēnjù

the conduit/network doctrine guides the theoretical basis

what theoretical basis?

针	灸	治疗
zhēn	jiǔ	zhìliáo

(that) of acupuncture and moxa therapy

Adjunct statement

这 是	不全面的
zhè shì	bùqúanmiànde

that is an incomplete (assumption)

<u>Second unit of meaning</u>

Statement

中	医	从来	没 有 脱离
zhōng	yī	cónglái	méi **yǒu** tuōlí

Chinese medicine **has** as yet not disassociated (itself)

from what?

范畴
fànchóu

from a realm (of thought)

from which realm of thought?	以 yǐ	经 jīng	络 luò	学说 xuéshuō	为 wéi	指导 zhǐdǎo	的 de

from one **taking** the conduit/network doctrine as   a guide

all Chinese medicine?	各 科 gè kē

all specialties

namely?	无论 wúlùn	内 科, nèi kē,

regardless whether it is the internal specialty, ...

以及 yǐjí	正 骨 zhèng gǔ

or   ... and setting bones

Third unit of meaning

Basic statement	重要性 zhòngyàoxìng

the importance (is obvious from the following)

what importance?	经 jīng	络 luò	学说 的 xuéshuō de

(that) **of** the conduit and network   doctrine

why is it obvious?	已经 证明 yǐjīng zhèngmíng

    a.)   it has already demonstrated (something)

what?

其 实际 价值
qí shíjì jiàzhí

its practical value

when?

在 长时期 实践 中
zài chángshíqí shíjiàn zhōng

during a longtime application

也 证实了 好些 问题
yě **zhèngshíle** hǎoxiē wèntí

b.)

it **has** also **provided evidence** to many questions

in what way?

初步
chūbù

preliminarily

when?

近来
jìnlái

recently

how?

通过 密切 合作
tōngguò mìqiè hézuò

through close cooperation

of whom with whom?

中 西 医
zhōng xī yī

of Chinese and Western medicine

where?

在 实验 研究 中
zài shíyàn yánjiū zhōng

in experimental research

81

Fourth unit of meaning

Basic statement

蠕动 ...	有	变化
rúdòng ...	yǒu	biànhuà

the peristalsis and ... undergo changes

what peristalsis?

胃	的
wèi	**de**

(that) **of** the stomach

what kind of
changes?

显明
xiǎnmíng

significant (ones)

when?

针刺	后
zhēncì	**hòu**

after needling

what?

委中	内庭	足 三里	等	穴
wěizhōng	nèitíng	zú sānlǐ	děng	xuè

the weizhong, neiting and leg sanli   holes

Adjunct statement

针刺	可	使
zhēncì	kě	shǐ

needling can cause (something)

needling what?

合谷，	三阴交	等	穴
hégǔ,	sānyīnjiāo	děng	xuè

the hegu and sanyinjiao   holes

what can it cause?

加强	和	间隔	缩短
jiāqiáng	hé	jiāngé	suōduǎn

a strengthening and an interval shortening

strengthening and
shortening of what?

子宫	收缩
zǐgōng	shōusuō

of uterus contractions

Fifth unit of meaning

Basic statement

这些	不	但	说明了	影响
zhèxiē	bù	dàn	shuōmíngle	yǐngxiǎng

these (effects) not only explain   the influence

which influence?

针刺	对	活动	的
zhēncì	duì	huódòng	de

(that) **of** needling on the activities

which activities?

内	脏
nèi	zāng

(those) of the internal depots

but?

也	说明了	关系
yě	shuōmíngle	guānxì

they also explain   relationships

which relationships?

经	络	与	脏	器	的
jīng	luò	yǔ	zāng	qì	de

(those) **of** the conduits/network with the depot-organs

83

Adjunct statement

值得	注意
zhídé	zhùyì

(that) is worth   attention

LESSON 4: PHYSIOLOGY

Text 4.1

Sentence structures

<u>First unit of meaning</u>

Basic statement

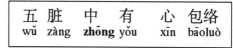

五　脏　是　心，　肝,...
wǔ　zàng　shì　xīn,　gān,...

the five depots are the heart, the liver...

1. Adjunct statement: structure identical with Basic statement

2. Adjunct statement

五　脏　中　有　心　包络
wǔ　zàng　**zhōng**　yǒu　xīn　bāoluò

among the five depots　　is　the heart enclosure

3. Adjunct statement

为　外　卫
wéi　wài　wèi

it is　the outer protection

what outer
protection?

心　的
xīn　**de**

(that) **of** the heart

4. Adjunct statement

有　　独立　起来
yǒu　　**dúlì**　qǐlái

it happens: (we)　　set up (something) **individually**

what?

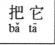

把它
bǎ　tā

it

5. Adjunct statement

列
liè

it is listed

how?

与 五 脏 并
yǔ wǔ zàng bìng

with the five depots together

6. Adjunct statement

称 为 六 脏
chēng wéi lìu zàng

they are designated as the six depots

7. Adjunct statement

功能 和 病 变 是 一致的
gōngnéng hé bìng biàn shì yīzhìde

functions and pathological changes are identical

which functions and pathological changes?

心 包络 的
xīn bāoluò de

(those) of the heart enclosure

identical with what?

与 心脏 相
yǔ xīnzàng xiāng

with the heart

Second unit of meaning

Basic statement

脏 和 腑 为 内 脏
zàng hé fǔ wéi nèi zàng

depots and palaces are inner depots

86

1. Adjunct statement

其　区别　是
qí　qūbié　shì

their difference is　(as follows)

2. Adjunct statement

五　脏　藏　精　气而　不泻
wǔ　zàng　cáng　jīng　qì ér　bú xiè

the five depots store essential qi　and do not drain

3. Adjunct statement: structure identical with 2.Adjunct statement

Third unit of meaning

Basic statement

凡　脏器　归属　于　　腑
fán　zàngqì　guīshǔ yú　　fǔ

all　organs belong to　the palaces

which organs?

具有的
jùyǒude

(those) having

having what?

功能
gōngnéng

(specific) functions

which functions?

出　　纳　　　　转输
chū　　nà　　　　zhuǎnshū

a.)　　　　they emit and take in and (thereby) forward

传　　化　　水　　谷
chuán　　huà　　shuǐ　　gǔ

b.)　　　　they transmit and transform water and grain

Adjunct statement

脏器 属 于 脏
zàngqì shǔ yú zàng

the organs belong to the depots

which organs?

没 有(的)
méi yǒu(de)

a.) (those) not having (something)

具有...的
jùyǒu...de

b.) (those) having (something)

what do they have/
have not

功能
gōngnéng

a function

which function?

直接 传 化
zhíjiē chuán huà

a.) (that of) directly transmitting and transforming

what?

水 谷
shuǐ gǔ

water and grain

贮藏
zhùcáng

b.) (that of) storing

what?

精 气
jīng qì

essential qi

88

Text 4.2

Sentence structures

<u>First unit of meaning</u>

Basic statement

心　生　　　血
xīn　shēng　　xuè

the heart generates the blood

Adjunct statement

(心)　主　　　藏　　神
(xīn)　zhǔ　　　cáng　shén

(the heart) is responsible for storing the spirit

<u>Second unit of meaning</u>

Statement

(心)　为　　主宰
(xīn)　wéi　zhǔzǎi

(the heart) is　the ruler

what ruler?

人　体　生命　　活动　　的
rén　tǐ　shēngmìng huódòng **de**

(that) **of** the human body's vital　　acitivities

<u>Third unit of meaning</u>

Statement

心脏 会　　　　　出现
xīnzàng huì　　　　chūxiàn

the heart　can let (something) appear

what?

症
zhèng

pathoconditions

which
pathoconditions?

心悸 ...　　或 谵 语 　等
xīnjì ...　　huò zhān yǔ 　děng

palpitation ... or 　wild talk ...

when?

本身　 不 健全
běnshēn　 bú jiànquán

(when) it itself 　 is not sound

why?

或　　　　受
huò　　　　shòu

a.)

either because it has received something

what?

情志的 刺激
qíngzhìde cìjī

an emotional stimulus

或 因　　 侵犯
huò yīn　　 qīnfàn

b.)

or 　because of an intrusion

intrusion of what?

病　　 邪 的
bìng　　 xié **de**

of a pathological evil

Fourth unit of meaning

Statement

心脏　 有了 病　　 变
xīnzàng　 yǒule bìng　　 biàn

the heart 　 has had 　 a pathological change

90

what happens?

本身 无　　以 自 主
běnshēn **wú**　　yǐ zì zhǔ

a.) it itself **has nothing** for self control

能 影响 活动
néng yǐngxiǎng huódòng

b.) it can influence activities

which activities?

其它 脏　　腑 的
qítā zàng　fǔ de

(those) **of** the other depots and palaces

Adjunct statement

使 之 发生 紊乱
shǐ zhī fāshēng wěnluàn

c.) it lets them develop disorder

Fifth unit of meaning

Basic statement

肝 藏　　血
gān cáng　xuè

the liver stores the blood

Adjunct statement

主　　谋 虑
zhǔ　　móu lü

it is responsible for plotting and planning

Sixth unit of meaning

Basic statement

肝 性 刚强
gān xìng gāngqiáng

the liver's nature is strength

1. Adjunct statement

故　　有　称号
gù　　yǒu　chēnghào

hence it has a designation

which designation?

将军　的
jiāngjūn　de

(that) of "general"

2. Adjunct statement

当　　　　受到　时
dāng　　　shòudào shí

when (the liver) receives　　(something)

receives what?

精神　刺激
jīngshén cìjī

mental　stimuli

what happens?

影响　其 功能　而　发生　症
yǐngxiǎng qí gōngnéng ér fāshēng zhèng

this influences its functions and generates pathoconditions

which functions?

正常
zhèngcháng

the normal　　　(functions)

which
pathoconditions?

恼怒　头 胀　　等
nǎonù　　tóu zhàng　děng

anger and head distention

3. Adjunct statement

火 气 上逆 而 发生　　吐 血
huǒ qì shàngnì ér fāshēng　tù xuè

the fire qi rises　and generates: one spits blood

always?

甚	至
shèn	zhì

in severe cases it goes so far

Seventh unit of meaning

Basic statement

肝	为	"先	天"
gān	wéi	"xiān	tiān"

the liver is   the "earlier dependence"

whose "earlier
dependence"?

女子	的
nüzǐ	**de**

(that) **of** women

1. Adjunct statement

有...的	意思
yǒu...**de**	yìsī

(this) has   the meaning **of** ...

of what?

生殖	机能	在	内
shēngzhí	jīnéng	zài	nèi

reproductive functions exist inside the (liver)

2. Adjunct statement

故	必须	重视
gù	bìxū	zhòngshì

hence it is essential to emphasize (something)

what?

治疗
zhìliáo

a therapy

which therapy?

对...的
duì...de

one being directed

directed at what?

肝脏
gānzàng

at the liver

when?

调   经
tiáo   jīng

a.)   when regulating the (monthly) period

种子
zhòngzǐ

b.)   when (enhancing) the fertility

Text 4.3

Sentence structures

<u>First unit of meaning</u>

Basic statement

脾	统	血
pí	tǒng	xuè

the spleen rules the blood

Adjunct statement

主	运	化
zhǔ	yùn	huà

it governs transport and transformation

<u>Second unit of meaning</u>

Basic statement

主要	是	营养
zhǔyào	shì	yíngyǎng

most important is   nourishment

most important for
what?

维持	力量
wéichí	lìliang

to maintain strength

which strength?

生命	的
shēngmìng	de

(that) **of** (our) life

1. Adjunct statement

脾	能
pí	néng

the spleen can   do (something)

95

what?

消化 水 谷
xiāohuà shuǐ gǔ

it digests water and grain

2. Adjunct statement

运输 到 全 身
yùnshū dào quán shēn

it transports through the entire body

what?

精华
jīnghuá

the essence

which essence?

食物 的
shíwù de

(that) **of** the food

3. Adjunct statement

故 被 称
gù bèi chēng

hence it is designated

as what?

为 本
wéi běn

as the basis

the basis of what?

后 天 之
hòu tiān zhī

(that) **of** the "later dependence"

96

Third unit of meaning

Basic statement

倘	运	化		能力	不 足
tǎng	yùn	huà		nénglì	bù zú

if the transport and transformation power is not enough

power of what?

脾	的
pí	**de**

(that) **of** the spleen

what happens?

则	作	胀
zé	zuò	zhàng

then (this) causes distention

when?

食	后
shí	**hòu**

after the meals

Adjunct statement

引起	肌肉	消瘦		精神	疲乏
yǐnqǐ	jīròu	xiāoshòu		jīngshén	pífá

(this) leads to muscular emaciation and to mental fatigue

Fourth unit of meaning

Basic statement

脾	又	主
pí	yòu	zhǔ

the spleen is further responsible

for what?

运	化	水湿
yùn	huà	shuǐshī

it transports and transforms the liquids

97

1. Adjunct statement

症 状	(是) 所	致
zhèng zhuàng	(shì) suǒ	zhì

the patho- manifestations (are) **those which** arrive

why do
they arrive?

大多	由于	脾	弱
dàduǒ	yǒuyú	pí	ruò

mostly because of splenic weakness

which patho-
manifestations are
these?

水湿	停滞	的
shuǐshī	tíngzhì	**de**

(those) **of** liquid stagnation

for example?

如	肌肤	浮肿,	大便	泄泻
rú	jīfū	fúzhǒng,	dàbiàn	xièxiè

e.g., skin edema, diarrhea

2. Adjunct statement

因此	用	方法
yīncǐ	yòng	fāngfǎ

hence (we) use methods

which methods?

健	脾
jiàn	pí

(those that) strengthen the spleen

why?

利	湿
lì	shī

to free the dampness

Fifth unit of meaning

Basic statement

肺　主　　　气
fèi　zhǔ　　　qì

the lung rules the qi

Adjunct statement

司　　　　清　　　肃
sī　　　　qīng　　　sù

it controls the clear and lofty

Sixth unit of meaning

Basic statement

肺　气　　不　降
fèi　qì　　bú　jiàng

if the lung qi does not descend

what happens?

引起 咳嗽,　　　气喘
yǐnqǐ késòu,　　　qìchuǎn

(this) causes coughing and panting

how?

最　易
zuì　yì

most easily

Adjunct statement

见 少　　气
jiàn shǎo　　qì

(we) see diminished qi and

言语　低怯　无　力
yányǔ　dīqiè　wú　lì

that the speech is faint　and without strength

99

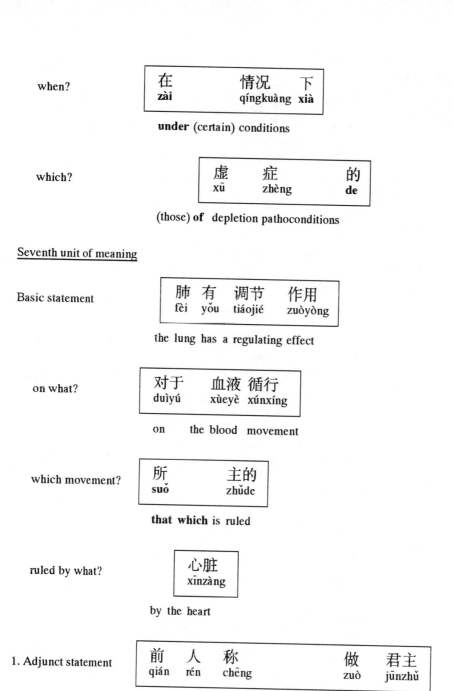

when?

在　　　情况　下
zài　qíngkuàng **xià**

under (certain) conditions

which?

虚　症　　的
xū　zhèng　**de**

(those) **of** depletion pathoconditions

Seventh unit of meaning

Basic statement

肺　有　调节　作用
fèi　yǒu　tiáojié　zuòyòng

the lung has a regulating effect

on what?

对于　　血液 循行
duìyú　xuèyè xúnxíng

on　the blood　movement

which movement?

所　　　主的
suǒ　zhǔde

that which is ruled

ruled by what?

心脏
xīnzàng

by the heart

1. Adjunct statement

前　人　称　　做　君主
qián　rén　chēng　zuò　jūnzhǔ

former people designated (something) as　the ruler

what?

心脏
xīnzàng

the heart

why?

为了 形容　　密切 关系
wèile xíngróng　mìqìe guānxì

to　　describe　the close　relationship

which relationship?

两者　间的
liǎngzhě **jiānde**

(that) **between** the two

2. Adjunct statement

称　　　作 相傅
chēng　zuò xiàngfù

they designated (something) as　minister

what?

肺脏
fèizàng

the lung

Text 4.4

Sentence structures

<u>First unit of meaning</u>

Basic statement

肾	藏	精
shèn	cáng	jīng

the kidneys store the essence

Adjunct statement

主	作	强
zhǔ	zuò	qiáng

they are responsible for generating strength

<u>Second unit of meaning</u>

Basic statement

肾脏	起有	积极	作用
shènzàng	qǐyǒu	jījí	zuòyòng

the kidneys develop a positive effect

on what?

对于	精力	充沛
duìyú	jīnglì	chōngpèi

on vigor abundance

on whose vigor
abundance?

人	的
rén	**de**

(on that) **of** man

Adjunct statement

肾	虚
shèn	xū

the kidneys are depleted

what happens?

则 症　　　　均 起
zé　zhèng　　　jūn qǐ

then pathoconditions do all　emerge

which
pathoconditions?

脑转,　　　耳 鸣
nǎozhuǎn,　ěr　míng

a.)

dizziness　and ear ringing

目 无　　　所　　　见,... 等
mù　wú　　　suǒ　　　jiàn,... děng

b.)

the eyes **have nothing** <u>by what</u> they see,...

Third unit of meaning

Basic statement

肾　为　"先　天"
shèn　wéi　"xiān　tiān"

the kidneys are　the "earlier dependence"

whose "earlier
dependence"?

男子 的
nánzǐ　**de**

(that) **of** males

1. Adjunct statement

与　　意义　相同
yǔ　　yìyì　**xiāngtóng**

(that) is **identical** with the meaning

the meaning of what?

以　　　肝 为　先　天　　　的
yǐ　　　gān wéi　xiān　tiān　　　**de**

(that) **of** considering the liver as　the "earlier dependence"

where?

女子
nǚzǐ

in females

2. Adjunct statement

指　　生殖　　功能　而　言
zhǐ　　shēngzhí　gōngnéng　ér　yán

(that) **refers** to reproductive functions

Fourth unit of meaning

Statement

症　　　　　　　从　　肾脏　治疗
zhèng　　　　　cóng　shènzàng　zhìliáo

pathoconditions are **treated** through the kidneys

which
pathoconditions?

性欲 衰退 及 滑　精,... 等
xìngyù shuāituì jí huá　jīng,... děng

libido decline and slipping semen, ...

Fifth unit of meaning

Basic statement

肾　有　特点
shèn　yǒu　tèdiǎn

the kidneys have a characteristic

which
characteristic?

一 不 同的
yī bù tóngde

one not identical

not identical
with what?

与　其它 内 脏
yǔ　qítā　nèi　zàng

with the other　inner depots

104

1. Adjunct statement

肾　有　两　枚
shèn　yǒu　liǎng méi

the kidneys have two   pieces

2. Adjunct statement

左者　为　　肾
zuǒzhě wéi　　shèn

the left　　is　　the kidney

3. Adjunct statement: structure identical with 2. Adjunct statement

4. Adjunct statement

肾　　主　　阴
shèn　zhǔ　　yīn

the kidney rules the yin

5. Adjunct statement: structure identical with 4. Adjunct statement

6. Adjunct statement

肾　　有　　称
shèn　yǒu　chēng

the kidneys have a designation

which designation?

脏　之
zàng　zhī

(that) of a depot

depot of what?

水　　火之
shuǐ　　huǒ zhī

(one) of water and fire

105

Text 4.5

Sentence structures

<u>First unit of meaning</u>

Basic statement

胆	为	腑
dǎn	wéi	fǔ

the gallbladder is   the palace

palace of what?

清净	之
qīngjìng	zhī

(that) **of** purity

Adjunct statement

主	决断
zhǔ	juéduàn

it rules decision making

<u>Second unit of meaning</u>

Basic statement

胆	与	肝	为 表	里
dǎn	yú	gān	wèi biǎo	lǐ

the gallbladder and the liver are outer and inner

1. Adjunct statement

肝	气	虽	强
gān	qì	suī	qiáng

the liver qi   may be strong

however?

非	胆	不 断
fēi	dǎn	bú duàn

if **there is no** gallbladder (it can) not decide

2. Adjunct statement

肝	胆	相	济
gān	dǎn	xiāng	**jì**

the liver and the gallbladder **provide** mutual **help**

what happens?

勇敢	乃	成
yǒnggǎn	**nǎi**	chéng

courage   forms **as a result**

Third unit of meaning

Basic statement

心	为	"君	火"
xīn	wéi	"jūn	huǒ"

the heart is   the "ruler fire"

which heart?

人	身
rén	shēn

(that in) the human body

1. Adjunct statement

胆	与	命	门	为	"相	火"
dǎn	yǔ	mìng	mén	wéi	"xiàng	huǒ"

gallbladder and life   gate   are   the "minister fire"

2. Adjunct statement

胆	火	偏	亢
dǎn	huǒ	piān	kàng

the gallbladder fire is unilaterally excessive

what happens?

则	出现	症
zé	chūxiàn	zhèng

then (this) produces pathoconditions

which
pathoconditions?

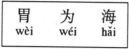

急躁	易	怒 ...	等
jízào	yì	nù ...	děng

restlessness and easily being angry, ...

Fourth unit of meaning

Basic statement

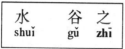

胃	为	海
wèi	wéi	hǎi

the stomach is   the sea

which sea?

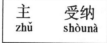

水	谷	之
shuǐ	gǔ	zhī

(that) of water and grain

Adjunct statement

主	受纳
zhǔ	shòunà

it rules the intake

Fifth unit of meaning

Basic statement

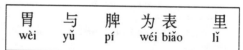

胃	与	脾	为表	里
wèi	yǔ	pí	wéi biǎo	lǐ

the stomach and the spleen are outer and inner

1. Adjunct statement

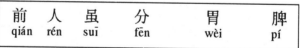

前	人	虽	分	胃	脾
qián	rén	suī	fēn	wèi	pí

earlier people may have differentiated stomach and spleen

in what regard?

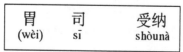

胃	司	受纳
(wèi)	sī	shòunà

a.)   (the stomach) controls the intake

108

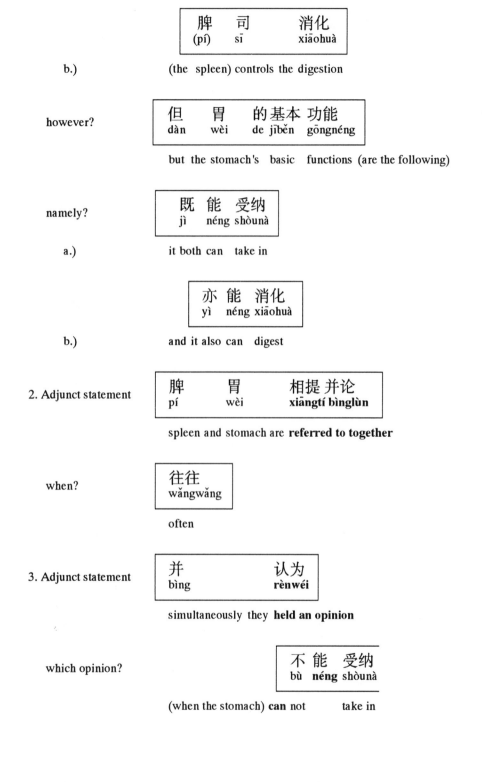

	脾	司	消化
	(pí)	sī	xiāohuà

b.) (the spleen) controls the digestion

however?

但	胃	的基本	功能
dàn	wèi	de jībĕn	gōngnéng

but the stomach's basic functions (are the following)

namely?

既	能	受纳
jì	néng	shòunà

a.) it both can take in

亦	能	消化
yì	néng	xiāohuà

b.) and it also can digest

2. Adjunct statement

脾	胃	相提 并论
pí	wèi	**xiāngtí bìnglùn**

spleen and stomach are **referred to together**

when?

往往
wǎngwǎng

often

3. Adjunct statement

并	认为
bìng	**rènwéi**

simultaneously they **held an opinion**

which opinion?

不	能	受纳
bù	**néng**	shòunà

(when the stomach) **can** not take in

就	谈不到	消化
jìu	tánbùdào	xiāohuà

then **there can be no talk of** digestion

Text 4.6

Sentence structures

<u>First unit of meaning</u>

Basic statement

小	肠	为	腑
xiǎo	cháng	wéi	fǔ

the small intestine is   the palace

which palace?

受	盛	之
shòu	shèng	**zhī**

(that) **of** receiving abundance

Adjunct statement

主	化	物
zhǔ	huà	wù

it is responsible for transforming things

<u>Second unit of meaning</u>

Basic statement

小	肠	承受	水	谷
xiǎo	cháng	chéngshòu	shuǐ	gǔ

the small intestine receives   water and grain

of which kind?

腐熟的
fǔshúde

decomposed (ones)

where have they
been decomposed?

胃	中
wèi	**zhōng**

in the stomach

111

1. Adjunct statement

进一步	分别	清	浊
jìnyíbù	fēnbié	qīng	zhuó

furthermore it separates the clear from the turbid

2. Adjunct statement

使
shǐ

it causes (something)

what?

精华	归	于	五	脏
jīnghuá	guī	yú	wǔ	zàng

a.)　　that the essence turns to　the five depots

what for?

贮藏
zhùcáng

for storage

b.: structure identical with a.

将	水液	归	于	膀胱
jiāng	shuǐyè	guī	yú	pángguāng

c.)　　it lets　the liquids turn to　the bladder

which liquids?

糟粕	中的
zāopò	**zhōngde**

(those) **being in** the waste

渣滓	归	于	大	肠
zhāzǐ	guī	yú	dà	cháng

d.)　　(it lets) the solid dregs turn to　the large intestine

Third unit of meaning

Statement

这些 都 是 工作
zhèxiē dōu shì gōngzuò

these all are functions

whose functions?

小 肠 的
xiǎo cháng **de**

(those) **of** the small intestine

to achieve what?

化 物
huà wù

to transform things

Fourth unit of meaning

Basic statement

大 肠 为 府
dà cháng wéi fǔ

the large intestine is the palace

which palace?

传导 之
chuándǎo **zhī**

(that) **of** transmission

Adjunct statement

主 排泄
zhǔ páixiè

it is responsible for excretion

Fifth unit of meaning

Basic statement

大	肠	接受	小	肠	糟粕
dà	cháng	jiēshòu	xiǎo	cháng	zāopò

the large intestine receives the small intestine's waste

1. Adjunct statement

负责	输送	排泄
fùzé	shūsòng	páixiè

it **is in charge of** transport and excretion

2. Adjunct statement

为	最后	阶段
wéi	zuìhòu	jiēduàn

it represents the very last phase

the very last phase of what?

整个	消化	过程	的
zhěnggè	xiāohuà	guòchéng	**de**

(that) **of** the entire digestion process

Sixth unit of meaning

Basic statement

凡	大便 闭结	着手
fán	dàbiàn bìjié	zhuóshǒu

each constipation ... is dealt with

how?

从	大	肠
cóng	dà	cháng

starting from the large intestine

why?

由于	功能	是	传导	职司
yóuyú	gōngnéng	shì	chuándǎo	zhísī

because the function is to transmit and to manage

114

what function?

大 肠 的
dà cháng **de**

(that) **of** the large intestine

to transmit what?

糟粕
zāopò

the waste

to manage what?

大便
dàbiàn

stools

Adjunct statement

有 不同的疗 法
yǒu bùtóngde liáo fǎ

there are different therapy patterns

namely?

通导, 润泽, 固 涩 等
tōngdǎo, rùnzé, gù sè děng

purging, moistening, and securing astriction

115

Text 4.7

Sentence structures

<u>First unit of meaning</u>

Basic statement

膀胱　为　官
pángguāng wéi guān

the bladder　is　the official

which official?

州　都　之
zhōu dū **zhī**

(that) **of** "Regional Rectifier"

Adjunct statement

司　气 化
sī qì huà

it controls the qi　transformation

<u>Second unit of meaning</u>

Basic statement

膀胱　为　处
pángguāng wéi chù

the bladder　is　the place

which place?

水液 潴汇 之
shuǐyè zhūhuì **zhī**

(that) **of** liquid　gathering

1. Adjunct statement

气 化　不 利
qì huà bù lì

the qi　transformation is not free

116

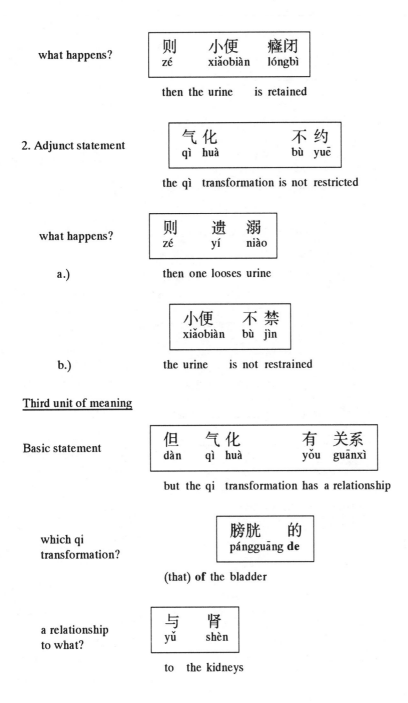

what happens?

则	小便	癃闭
zé	xiǎobiàn	lóngbì

then the urine is retained

2. Adjunct statement

气 化	不 约
qì huà	bù yuē

the qì transformation is not restricted

what happens?

则	遗	溺
zé	yí	niào

a.)   then one looses urine

小便	不	禁
xiǎobiàn	bù	jìn

b.)   the urine is not restrained

Third unit of meaning

Basic statement

但	气 化	有	关系
dàn	qì huà	yǒu	guānxì

but the qi transformation has a relationship

which qi
transformation?

膀胱	的
pángguāng	de

(that) of the bladder

a relationship
to what?

与	肾
yǔ	shèn

to the kidneys

1. Adjunct statement

肾	气	足
shèn	qì	zú

the kidney qi is sufficient

what happens?

则		能	化
zé		néng	huà

then (the bladder) can transform (qi)

2. Adjunct statement: structure identical with 1. Adjunct statement

3. Adjunct statement

治	小便	不利	或 不禁
zhì	xiǎobiàn	bùlì	huò bùjìn

(we) treat urine   that is impeded or unrestrained

what happens?

有时		应	用	法
yǒushí		yīng	yòng	fǎ

sometimes (we) should use a pattern

which pattern?

温	肾	之
wēn	shèn	zhī

(that) **of** warming the kidneys

Fourth unit of meaning

Basic statement

三	焦	为	官
sān	jiāo	wéi	guān

the triple burner is the official

which official?

决	渎	之
jué	dú	zhī

(that) **of** clearing the ditches

118

Adjunct statement

主	行	水
zhǔ	xíng	shuǐ

it is responsible for transmitting water

Fifth unit of meaning

Statement

三	焦	组成
sān	jiāo	zǔchéng

the triple burner is composed

of what?

由 三	部分
yóu sān	bùfēn

of three parts

which are they?

上 焦,	中 焦,	下 焦
shàng jiāo,	zhōng jiāo,	xià jiāo

upper burner, central burner, lower burner

Sixth unit of meaning

Basic statement

它 的作用	为	疏通	水 道
tā de zuòyòng	wéi	shūtōng	shuǐ dào

its function is to dredge the water ways

1. Adjunct statement

例如	治	胀	满
lìrú	zhì	zhàng	mǎn

e.g., (we) treat swelling and fullness

which swelling and fullness?

停	水
tíng	shuǐ

(those resulting from) stagnating water

what happens?

用 利　　　气
yòng lì　　　qì

(we) **use** stimulating the qi (flow)

why?

来 帮助　　行　　　水
lái bāngzhú　xíng　　shuǐ

to assist　in transmitting the water

3. Adjunct statement

用　　药物
yòng　yàowù

(we) employ drugs

which drugs?

疏畅的
shūchàngde

opening　(ones)

what do they open?

三　焦
sān　jiāo

the triple burner

when are they employed?

所谓 利　　　气
suǒwèi lì　　　qì

for the so-called stimulating the qi (flow)

120

Text 4.8

Sentence structures

<u>First unit of meaning</u>

Basic statement

有	奇恒之	腑
yǒu	qíhéngzhī	fǔ

there are extraordinary palaces

in what regard?

脏	腑	之外
zàng	fǔ	**zhīwài**

in addition to the depots and palaces

Adjunct statement

即	脑,	髓,	骨,	脉, ...
jí	nǎo,	suǐ,	gǔ,	mài, ...

these are the brain, the marrow, the bones, the vessels, ...

<u>Second unit of meaning</u>

Basic statement

意义	是
yìyì	shì

the meaning is (the following)

the meaning of what?

奇恒	的
qíhéng	**de**

(that) **of** "extraordinary"

1. Adjunct statement

似	脏	非	脏
sì	zàng	**fēi**	zàng

they resemble depots but they **are not** depots

2. Adjunct statement: structure identical with 1. Adjunct statement

121

3. Adjunct statement

形 虽 似　　府
xíng suī sì　　fǔ

the shape may resemble a palace

but?

而　　作用 似　　　　脏
ér　　zuòyòng sì　　　　zàng

but their function resembles (that of) a depot

4. Adjunct statement

是 一 种　　内 脏
shì yī zhǒng　　nèi zàng

they are a　type　of inner depot

which type?

异　　乎　　寻常的
yì　　hū　　xúnchángde

different　　from normal　　(ones)

Third unit of meaning

Statement

它们 是 部分
tāmen shì bùfēn

they　are parts

what kind of parts?

极其 重要的
jíqí　zhòngyàode

very　important　(ones)

where?

在　　人 体 中
zài　　rén tǐ zhōng

inside the human body

122

Fourth unit of meaning

Basic statement

这些	府	并不 是	孤立的
zhèxiē	fǔ	**bìngbù** shì	gūlìde

these   palaces   are **by no means** isolated

which palaces?

奇恒之
qíhéngzhī

(these) extraordinary (ones)

1. Adjunct statement

都 有	联系
dōu yǒu	liánxì

they all have a relationship

to what?

和	脏	腑
hé	zàng	fǔ

to   the depots and palaces

2. Adjunct statement

比如	脑	和	心	肝	有	关系
bǐrú	nǎo	hé	xīn	gān	yǒu	guānxì

e.g.,   brain and heart/ liver have a relationship

3. Adjunct statement

髓	和	骨	有	关
suǐ	hé	gǔ	yǒu	guān

marrow and bones have a relationship

why?

因	脑	和	髓	有	关
yīn	nǎo	hé	suǐ	yǒu	guān

because brain and marrow have a relationship

4. Adjunct statement

骨　属　于　肾
gǔ　shǔ　yú　shèn

the bones belong to　the kidneys

5. Adjunct statement: structure identical with 3. Adjunct statement

6. Adjunct statement

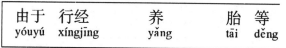

女子胞 即　　子宫　属　　　肝
nǚzǐbāo　jí　　zǐgōng　shǔ　　gān

the womb　　is　the uterus, it belongs to the liver

7. Adjunct statement

由于　行经　　　养　　胎　等
yóuyú　xíngjīng　　yǎng　　tāi　děng

because menstruation and nourishing the fetus

有　关
yǒu　guān

have a relationship

to what?

与　血
yǔ　xuè

to　the blood

hence?

故　　又 有 关
gù　　yòu yǒu guān

hence they also have a relationship

to what?

和 心　脾
hé xīn　pí

to　heart and spleen

124

Fifth unit of meaning

Basic statement

还	有	府
hái	**yǒu**	fǔ

also **there are** palaces

what kind of palaces?

传	化	之
chuán	huà	**zhī**

(those) **of** transmission and transformation

what are they like?

与	奇恒之	府	对称的
yǔ	qíhéngzhī	fǔ	**duìchēngde**

symmetric to   the extraordinary palaces

1. Adjunct statement

即	胃,	大	肠
jí	wèi,	dà	cháng, ...

these are the stomach, the large intestine, ...

2. Adjunct statement

这	五个	腑	属	于	消化	系统
zhè	wǔge	fǔ	shǔ	yú	xiāohuà	xìtǒng

these five   palaces belong to   the digestive system

where?

在	六	腑	中
zài	lìu	fǔ	**zhōng**

among the six   palaces

Sixth unit of meaning

Basic statement

如	所	述
rú	**suǒ**	shù

it is like **that which** was said

where?

上
shàng

above

Adjunct statement

联系　　是 完整的　　不 可分离的
liánxì　　shì wánzhěngde　　bù kěfēnlíde

the relationships are integrated　　and not divisible

which
relationships?

都是 有机的
dōushì yǒujíde

all　　organic (ones)

which relationships?

全　身　组织
quán shēn zǔzhī

(those) of the entire body structure

126

LESSON 5: BLOOD AND QI

Text 5.1

Sentence structures

<u>First unit of meaning</u>

Basic statement

气	和	血	并	重
qì	hé	xuè	bìng	zhòng

qi and blood are equally important

1. Adjunct statement

作		为	统帅
zuò		wéi	tǒngshuài

(we) consider (something) as commander

what?

气
qì

the qi

as commander of what?

血	的
xuè	**de**

(as that) **of** the blood

2. Adjunct statement

这	是	一种	认识	方法
zhè	shì	yīzhǒng	rènshí	fāngfǎ

this is a cognitive pattern

where?

生理	上的
shēnglǐ	**shàngde**

(one) **being** in the physiology

127

in which physiology?

中　医
zhōng　yī

(in that) of Chinese medicine

Second unit of meaning

Basic statement

名称　　　相当　多
míngchēng　xiāngdāng duō

the designations are quite　　numerous

which designations?

气 的
qì　de

(those) **of** qi

1. Adjunct statement

有　　　元　气，　真　气，...
yǒu　　yuán　qì,　zhēn qì, ...

there are the original qi,　the true　qi, ...

2. Adjunct statement

这些 都是 指　气　血
zhèxiē dōushì zhǐ　qì　xuè

they　all　refer to qi　and blood

和 其它 物质　　及 能力
hé qítā　wùzhì　jí nénglì

and other　substances and abilities

where?

整个 人 体 内
zhěnggè rén　tǐ　**nèi**

in the entire　human body

128

3. Adjunct statement

名 虽 异 而
míng **suī** yì ér

the names **may be** different, and yet

实 为 一种
shí wéi yīzhǒng

the facts are identical

Third unit of meaning

Basic statement

另 有 称
lìng **yǒu** chēng

besides, **there are** designations

which?

阳 气, 阴 气之
yáng qì, yīn qì **zhī**

(those) **of** yang qi   and yin qi

1. Adjunct statement

这 是
zhè shì

that is (to serve the following purpose)

namely?

分别 两 大 作用
fēnbié liǎng dà zuòyòng

to distinguish two   major functions

where?

从 元 气内
cóng yuán qì **nèi**

from **within** the original qi

2. Adjunct statement

（这）说明
(zhè) shuōmíng

(they) explain   (something)

what?

一 种　　能 保卫 体 表
yī zhǒng　néng bǎowéi tǐ biǎo

a.)

one type   (of qi) can protect the body's exterior

另一 种 能 保持 精力　不使 亏耗
lìngyī zhǒng néng bǎochí jīnglì　bùshǐ kuīhào

b.)

another type can conserve vigor and prevent loss

3. Adjunct statement

故　　叫 真 阳,　真 阴
gù　　jiào zhēn yáng,　zhēn yīn

hence they are called true yang and true yin

Fourth unit of meaning

Basic statement

有 宗 气,　中 气
yǒu zòng qì,　zhōng qì

there are ancestral qi   and central qi

1. Adjunct statement

指
zhǐ

they refer (to something)

to what?

有 一 部分
yǒu yī bùfèn

there is one part

130

where?

元　气中
yuán　qì zhōng

in the original qi

2. Adjunct statement

属　于　上　焦　　肺
shǔ　yú　shàng jiāo　fèi

it belongs to　the upper burner and the lung

3. Adjunct statement

另一 部分 属　于　中　焦 ...
lìngyī bùfèn shǔ　yú　zhōng jiāo ...

another part　belongs to　the central burner, ...

4. Adjunct statement

所以　　叫 肺 气,　胃　气
suǒyǐ　jiào fèi qì,　wèi　qì

hence they are called lung qi　and stomach qi

Fifth unit of meaning

Statement

概括的 说　　均 为 元　气
gàikuòde shuō　jūn wéi yuán　qì

generally speaking, they all are original qi

131

Text 5.2

Sentence structures

<u>First unit of meaning</u>

Basic statement

气 代表　能力,…　物质
qì　dàibiǎo　nénglì,…　wùzhì

qi　represents power, …　substance

which qi?

气　　血　的
qì　　xuè　**de**

(that) **of** qi　and blood

where?

有些 地方
yǒuxiē dìfāng

(at) some　places

Adjunct statement

因而 有　　　说法
yīn'ér **yǒu**　　shuōfǎ

hence **there is** an opinion

which opinion?

气 属　　　　无　形
qì　shǔ　　　　<u>wú</u>　xíng

(that) **of** "qi　belongs to (that which) <u>has</u> <u>no</u> form

血 为　　有 形 的
xuè　wéi　　yǒu xíng **de**

blood is (that which) has　form"

Second unit of meaning

Basic statement

我们的 体会
wǒmende tǐhuì

(it is) our   understanding

1. Adjunct statement

前　人　提出
qián　rén　tíchū

earlier people proposed (something)

what?

把 气 和 血　　　对待
bǎ qì hé xuè　　　duìdài

to treat   qi and blood (as follows)

2. Adjunct statement

血　是 物质
xuè　shì wùzhì

blood is   substance

3. Adjunct statement

气 应该 是 物质
qì yīnggāi shì wùzhì

the qi   should be substance

4. Adjunct statement

作用　是 "能力"
zuòyòng shì "nénglì"

the effect   is   "power"

which effect?

气 所　　　发生的
qì suǒ　　　fāshēngde

that which is brought forth by the <u>qi</u>

133

Third unit of meaning

Basic statement

血液 循行　　　　脉　内
xuèyè xúnxíng　　　mài　nèi

the blood　moves　**inside** the vessels

1. Adjunct statement

全　身　受　其营养
quán shēn shòu　qí yíngyǎng

the entire body receives its　nourishment

2. Adjunct statement

气 能 改善 和 帮助
qì　néng gǎishàn hé　bāngzhú

the qi　can　improve and assist

what can it
improve?

功能
gōngnéng

ability

what can it
assist?

正常　　运行
zhèngcháng yùnxíng

the normal　　movement

what ability and
movement?

血液 的
xuèyè de

(those) **of** the blood

3. Adjunct statement

二者 是 重要　因素
èrzhě　shì zhòngyào yīnsù

both　are important elements

elements of which kind?

| 构成....的 |
| gòuchéng....de |

(those) generating (something)

what?

| 正常 | 生理 | 活动 |
| zhèngcháng | shēnglǐ | huódòng |

normal   physiological activities

which activities?

| 人 | 体 |
| rén | tǐ |

(those of the) human body

4. Adjunct statement

| (二者) | 是 | 绝对 | 不 | 能分离的 |
| (èrzhě) | shì | juéduì | bù | néngfēnlíde |

(both)   are definitely not separable

Fourth unit of meaning

Basic statement

| 假使 | 气 | 受到 | 刺激 |
| jiǎshǐ | qì | shòudào | cìjī |

if   the qi   receives stimuli

which stimuli?

| 心理上(的) | 环境上的 |
| xīnlǐshàng(de) | huánjìngshàngde |

psychological or environmental (ones)

what will
happen?

| 都 | 会 | 影响 | 到 | 血 |
| dōu | huì | yǐngxiǎng | dào | xuè |

all can exert an influence on the blood

who exerts an
influence?

无论	喜,	乐
wúlùn	xǐ,	lè

a.)

regardless whether it is happiness, ... or joy

what stimuli are they?

情志	方面的
qíngzhì	**fāngmiànde**

(those) **concerning** the emotions

冷	热
lěng	rè

b.)

or cold and heat

what stimuli are they?

气候	方面的
qìhòu	**fāngmiànde**

those **concerning** the climate

劳	逸
láo	yì

c.)

or fatigue and idleness

what stimuli are they?

工作	方面的
gōngzuò	**fāngmiànde**

those **concerning** work

Fifth unit of meaning

Basic statement

前	人	重视	气
qián	rén	zhòngshì	qì

earlier people emphasized the qi

136

1. Adjunct statement

称做	"气	为	血	帅"
chēngzuò	"qì	wéi	xuè	shuài"

they stated   "the qi is the blood commander"

2. Adjunct statement

说	"百	病	皆	生	于	气"
shuō	"bǎi	bìng	jiē	shēng	yú	qì"

they said **"all** illnesses   emerge from the qi"

Text 5.3

Sentence structures

First unit of meaning

Basic statement

虽	当		用 血 分 药
suī	dāng		yòng xuè fèn yào

although it is appropriate to use   blood section drugs

what for?

治疗
zhìliáo

for treatment

when?

血	分	病
xuè	fèn	bìng

(in case of) blood section illness

but?

但还		有	治	法
dàn hái		yǒu	zhì	fǎ

but **in addition** <u>there</u> <u>are</u> therapy patterns

which therapy patterns?

a.)

理	气	和		血
lǐ	qì	hé		xuè

to regulate the qi   to harmonize the blood

b.)

行	气	逐	瘀
xíng	qì	zhú	yū

to move the qi   to eliminate stagnations

c.)

血	脱	益		气
xuè	tuō	yì		qì

in case of blood loss to increase the qi

138

1. Adjunct statement

这 是 因为
zhè shì yīnwèi

that is   because (of the following)

namely?

气 行 则 血 行
qì xíng zé xuè xíng

a.)   when the qi moves, then the blood moves

气 滞 则 血 滞
qì zhì zé xuè zhì

b.)   when the qi slackens, then the blood slackens

2. Adjunct statement

要 使
yào shǐ

(we) wish to cause (the following)

what?

血液 循行 正常
xuèyè xúnxíng zhèngcháng

(that) the blood flow is normal

what do we do?

先 使 气 机 舒畅
xiān shǐ qì jī shūchàng

first (we) cause the qi flow to be unimpeded

3. Adjunct statement

要 使
yào shǐ

(we) wish to cause (the following)

what?

瘀 血 排除
yū xuè páichú

the stagnating blood is eliminated

what does one do?

先	使	气 分	通利
xiān	shǐ	qì fèn	tōnglì

first (we) cause the qi   section to be passable

Second unit of meaning

Basic statement

还	能 用 药
hái	néng yòng yào

furthermore (we) can   use   drugs

which drugs?

补	气
bǔ	qì

(those which) supplement qi

why?

来 帮助	收摄
lái bāngzhù	shōushè

to   help   to acquire   (blood)

when?

在	症候
zài	zhènghòu

in the presence of symptoms

which symptoms?

出血	不	止 的
chūxuè	bù	zhǐ **de**

(those) **of** bleeding without end

Adjunct statement

同样	需要 用
tóngyàng	xūyào yòng

similarly, (we) must   use   (something)

140

what?	补　　　气 药 bǔ　　　qì yào	

drugs supplementing qi

why?	来 加速　恢复 lái jiāsù　huīfù

to　speed up recovery

on which basis?	根据　　道理 gēnjù　　dàolǐ

on the basis　of a principle

which principle?	阳 生 则　　阴 长 的 yáng shēng zé　　yīn zhǎng **de**

(that) **of** "when the yang lives　then the yin　grows"

when?	严重的　贫血 症 yánzhòngde pínxuè zhèng

in case of serious　　anemia pathoconditions

Third unit of meaning

Statement	这些 方法　都 是　很 有效的 zhèxiē fāngfǎ　**dōu** shì　hěn yǒuxiàode

these　procedures　　are **all** very effective (ones)

where?	在 临症　　上 **zài** línzhèng　　**shàng**

in　clinical　practice

Fourth unit of meaning

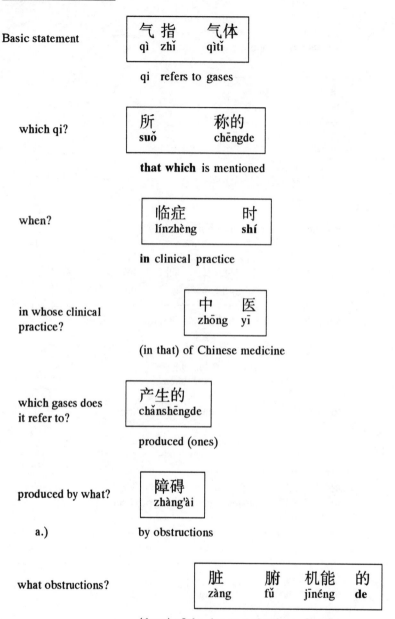

Basic statement

气 指　　气体
qì　zhǐ　　qìtǐ

qi　refers to gases

which qi?

所　　　　称的
suǒ　　　　chēngde

that which is mentioned

when?

临症　　　　时
línzhèng　　　shí

in clinical practice

in whose clinical practice?

中　　医
zhōng　yī

(in that) of Chinese medicine

which gases does it refer to?

产生的
chǎnshēngde

produced (ones)

produced by what?

障碍
zhàng'ài

a.)　　by obstructions

what obstructions?

脏　　腑　　机能　　的
zàng　　fǔ　　jīnéng　　de

(those) **of** the depots and palaces functions

或	消化	不 良 等
huò	xiāohuà	bù liáng děng

b.)　　　　　　　　or　when the digestion is not good

Fifth unit of meaning

Statement

用	名词
yòng	míngcí

(Chinese medicine) employs terms

which terms?

气 滞,	气 雍,	气 郁 ...	等
qì zhì,	qì yōng,	qì yù ...	děng

qi　sluggishness, qi　obstruction, qi　stagnation, ...

when does it use these terms?

常	见的
cháng	jiànde

(in case) of often　seen　(conditions)

for example?

如	胸 膈	痞	闷
rú	xiōng gé	pǐ	mèn

e.g., chest- diaphragm block and pressure

Adjunct statement

作	为 病理的	解释
zuò	wéi bìnglǐde	jiěshì

it turns them into pathological explanations

Sixth unit of meaning

Statement

用	气字	为病	名
yòng	qì zì	wéi bìng	míng

it uses the qi　character as　illness name

when?

多
duō

often

for example?

如 气 膈,　　和 肝 气 痛 等等
rú　qì　gé,　　hé　gān　qì ... tòng děngděng

e.g., qi　blockages, ... and liver qi ... pain and so forth

when?

病症
bìngzhèng

(in case of) illnesses

which illnesses?

发生的
fāshēngde

(those) bringing forth (something)

what do they
bring forth?

这些 症 状
zhèxiē zhèng zhuàng

these　patho- manifestations

144

Text 5.4

Sentence structures

<u>First unit of meaning</u>

Statement

全　身　都　靠　　　营养
quán　shēn　**dōu** kào　　　yíngyǎng

the **entire** body　　depends on nourishment

provided by what?

血液
xuèyè

(by) the blood

<u>Second unit of meaning</u>

Statement

凡是　　　心脏　衰弱　或　　血　亏
fánshì　　xīnzàng　shuāiruò huò　　xuè　kuī

whenever the heart　is weak　or　the blood is deficient

循行　失　调
xúnxíng　shǐ　tiáo

and when the movement loses its regular order

what is then?

会 出现
huì chūxiàn

(this) can bring forth (something)

namely?

心悸,　惊惕,　脉 来　歇止
xīnjì,　jìngtì,　mài lái　xiēzhǐ

palpitation, shock,　pulse arrival stop

145

Basic statement

血液 得 寒
xuèyè dé hán

the blood receives cold

what will happen?

则 凝 滞
zé níng zhì

then it congeals and slackens

1. Adjunct statement: structure identical with Basic statement

2. Adjunct statement

这 寒 和 热 包括
zhè hán hé rè bāokuò

this cold and this heat include (something)

what?

寒 邪 和 热 邪
hán xié hé rè xié

a.)   cold evil and heat evil

which cold and
heat evil?

外 界 的
wài jiè de

(those) of the external world

寒凉 和 辛 热
hánliáng hé xīn rè

b.)   coldness and acrid heat

which coldness and
acrid heat?

饮 食 的
yǐn shí de

(those) of beverages and food

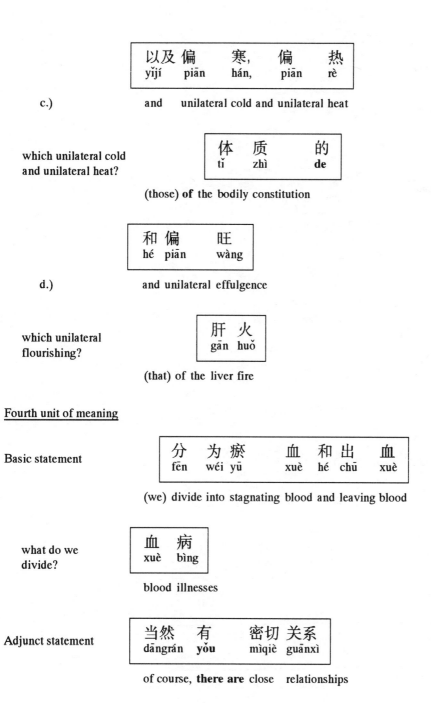

	以及	偏	寒,	偏	热
	yǐjí	piān	hán,	piān	rè

c.)   and   unilateral cold and unilateral heat

which unilateral cold
and unilateral heat?

体	质	的
tǐ	zhì	**de**

(those) **of** the bodily constitution

和	偏	旺
hé	piān	wàng

d.)   and unilateral effulgence

which unilateral
flourishing?

肝	火
gān	huǒ

(that) of the liver fire

Fourth unit of meaning

Basic statement

分	为	瘀	血	和	出	血
fēn	wéi	yū	xuè	hé	chū	xuè

(we) divide into stagnating blood and leaving blood

what do we
divide?

血	病
xuè	bìng

blood illnesses

Adjunct statement

当然	有	密切	关系
dāngrán	**yǒu**	mìqiè	guānxì

of course, **there are** close   relationships

to what?

与　气
yǔ　qì

to　the qi

Fifth unit of meaning

Basic statement

血　虚　起
xuè　xū　qǐ

blood depletion emerges

from what?

于　疲劳　过度
yú　píláo　guòdù

a.)　　from fatigue in excess

出血　过多
chūxuè　guòduō

b.)　　(from) bleeding excessively

what kind of bleeding?

创　伤
chuāng shāng

(that of) wound injuries

when?

病　后
bìng　**hòu**

a.)　　**after** illnesses

及　妇人　产　后
jí　fùrén　chǎn　**hòu**

b.)　　and in females **after** delivery

1. Adjunct statement

须	治疗
xū	zhìliáo

it is essential to treat

in what way?

从	三	脏
cóng	sān	zàng

starting from the three depots

which three depots?

心,	肝,	脾
xīn,	gān,	pí

heart, liver and spleen

when?

当	已经	成为	时
dāng	yǐjing	chéngwéi	**shí**

when (something) has already formed

what?

血	虚	症
xuè	xū	zhèng

a blood depletion pathocondition

2. Adjunct statement

应	治疗
yīng	zhìliáo

it is appropriate to treat

in what way?

从	肾脏
cóng	shènzàng

starting from the kidneys

when?

必要	时
bìyào	**shí**

when necessary

149

Text 5.5

Sentence structures

First unit of meaning

Statement

精	是	物质	基础
jīng	shì	wùzhì	jīchǔ

essence is   the material basis

of what?

生长,	发育	以及	生殖	能力	的
shēngzhǎng, fāyù		yǐjí	shēngzhí	nénglì	**de**

of growth,   development, and   reproductive power

what growth, ...?

人	体
rén	tǐ

(that) of the human body

Second unit of meaning

Basic statement

中	医	归		于	肾脏
zhōng	yī	guī		yú	shènzàng

Chinese medicine associates (something) with the kidneys

what?

精
jīng

essence

1. Adjunct statement

精	为	基础
jīng	wéi	jīchǔ

essence is   the basis

the basis of what?

生命　　的
shēngmìng **de**

(that) **of** life

2. Adjunct statement

所以　称　　肾
suǒyǐ　chēng　shèn

hence it designates the　kidneys

为　　"先　天"
wéi　"xiān　tiān"

as　the "earlier dependencies"

<u>Third unit of meaning</u>

Basic statement

靠　　饮　　食
kào　yǐn　shí

(it) depends on drink and food

what for?

来 给养
lái jǐyǎng

for nourishment

when?

待到　　出生　以后
dàidào　chūshēng **yǐhòu**

after　it was born

1. Adjunct statement

这 是　作用
zhè shì　zuòyòng

that is　the function

the function of what?	脾 pí	胃 wèi	的 **de**

(that) **of** spleen and stomach

2. Adjunct statement

故 gù		称 chēng	脾 pí	胃 wèi

hence (Chinese medicine) designates spleen and stomach

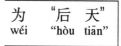

为 wéi	"后 天" "hòu tiān"

as the "later dependencies"

3. Adjunct statement

并 bìng		认为 rènwéi

simultaneously (Chinese medicine) believes (something)

in which context?

在 临症 **zài** línzhèng	上 **shàng**

in clinical practice

4. Adjunct statement

先 天 xiān tiān	不 足 bù zú

the earlier dependencies are not sufficient

what is then?

可 kě	用 yòng	后 天 hòu tiān

it is possible to use the later dependencies

what for?

来 调 lái tiáo	养 yǎng

to regulate the nourishment

152

Fourth unit of meaning

Basic statement

精　有　密切　影响
jīng　yǒu　mìqiè　yǐngxiǎng

essence has a close influence

on what?

对于　体　力
duìyú　tǐ　lì

on bodily strength

Adjunct statement

人　呈　腰　酸, 背　痛,
rén　chéng　yāo　suān, bèi　tòng, ...

persons present lumbar pain, back pain, ...

which persons?

患... 的
huàn...de

suffering (ones)

what do they
suffer from?

有　　　　遗　精
yǒu　　　　yí　jīng

they have (the problem) to lose semen

Fifth unit of meaning

Basic statement

由于　　肾　主　藏　精
yóuyú　　shèn　zhǔ　cáng　jīng

because the kidneys master storing essence

what has happened?

称　之　为肾　亏
chēng　zhī　wéi shèn　kuī

(we) designate them as kidney deficiency

153

<table>
<tr><td>what is desig-
nated as kidney
deficiency?</td><td>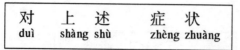</td></tr>
</table>

what is designated as kidney deficiency?

对　　上　述　　症　状
duì　　shàng shù　　zhèng zhuàng

the above mentioned patho- manifestations

when?

一般
yībān

generally

Adjunct statement

以　　补　　　　肾　　为主
yǐ　　bǔ　　　　shèn　　wéi zhǔ

(we) consider supplementing the kidneys as primary

Sixth unit of meaning

Basic statement

必须　　　指出
bìxū　　　zhǐchū

it is necessary to emphasize (something)

what?

有　　很　多　地方
yǒu　　hěn duō dìfāng

there are very many places

where?

中　　医　　书　上
zhōng　yī　　shū　shàng

in Chinese medical texts

**what do these
places do?**

指　　精
zhǐ　　jīng

they refer to essence

154

which essence?

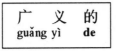

(one) **of** a broad sense

Adjunct statement

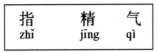

they refer to the essential qi

which essential qi?

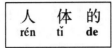

(that) **of** the human body

Seventh unit of meaning

Statement

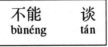

it is impossible to speak (about essence in a broad sense)

how?

confused into one

confused with what?

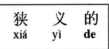

with the essence

with which essence?

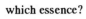

(that) **of** the narrow sense

155

Text 5.6

Sentence structures

<u>First unit of meaning</u>

Basic statement

前	人	认为
qián	rén	rènwéi

earlier people held (the following)

what?

各 组织	都	是	有形的
gè zǔzhī	**dōu**	shì	yǒuxíngde

all structures   are tangible

which structures?

人	体	的
rén	tǐ	**de**

(those) **of** the human body

1. Adjunct statement

还	有	一 种	能力
hái	**yǒu**	yī zhǒng	nénglì

also, **there** **is** a   kind of a power

which kind?

一个	高	级的,	无形的
yīge	gāo	jíde	wúxíngde

a   high ranking, shapeless (one)

where?

在	主持	活动
zài	zhǔchí	huódòng

in directing activities

156

2. Adjunct statement

称 它 为 "神"
chēng tā wéi "shén"

they designated this as "spirit"

Second unit of meaning

Basic statement

假使 神 能 充旺
jiǎshǐ shén néng chōngwàng

if the spirit faculties are complete

what is then?

内 脏 和 形 体 活泼
nèi zàng hé xíng tǐ huópō

the internal depots and the physical body are active

Adjunct statement

神 一 涣散
shén yī huànsǎn

as soon as the spirit slackens

what is then?

一切不 起 作用 了
yīqièbù qǐ zuòyòng le

none will fulfill its functions

Third unit of meaning

Basic statement

神 发生 病 变
shén fāshēng bìng biàn

the spirit exhibits pathological changes

Adjunct statement

会 产生
huì chǎnshēng

these can generate (something)

157

what?

症 状
zhèng zhuàng

patho-manifestations

which?

一　　系列 的
yī　　xìliè　de

(those) **of** a whole series

namely?

a.)

胸 膈　　烦　　　　闷
xiōng gé　　fán　　　　mèn

chest/diaphragm uneasiness and pressure

b.)

两 胁　　不 舒
liǎng xié　　bù shū

both flanks are not relaxed

c.)

精神　　不 能　　自 主
jīngshén　　bù néng　　zì zhǔ

the mind　　is not capable of self control

d.)

手　　足 无　　力
shǒu　　zú **wú**　　lì

hands and feet **have no** strength

e.)

狂妄　　　　不 识　　人
kuángwàng　　　　bù shí　　rén

(the patient) is frantic　　and does not recognize people

f.)

记忆 力　　衰退
jìyì　　lì　　shuāituì

(the patient's) memory strength weakens

前阴 萎缩
qiányīn wěisuō

g.)   the genitals shrink

腰	背 酸痛
yāo	bèi suāntòng

h.)   lumbar and back pain

不 能	俯	仰
bù néng	fǔ	yǎng

j.)   (the patient) is not able to lower or lift   (his/her head),

转	侧
zhuǎn	cè

or to turn   to the side

Fourth unit of meaning

Statement

丸 是 治疗的
wán shì zhìliáode

pills are curing (ones)

which pills?

如	朱砂	安	神	丸
rú	zhūshā	ān	shén	wán

a.)   e.g., the "cinnabar-pacifies-the-spirit" pills

琥珀 定	志 丸
hǔpò dìng	zhì wán

b.)   the "amber-stabilizes-the-will" pills

159

where are these pills?

成	方	中
chéng	fāng	**zhōng**

among the established prescriptions

what do they cure?

这	种	病
zhè	zhǒng	bìng

these kinds of illnesses

Fifth unit of meaning

Basic statement

神	不	是	空洞的
shén	bù	shì	kōngdòngde

the spirit is not   an empty (something)

Adjunct statement

需要	物质	来	营养
xūyào	wùzhì	lái	yíngyǎng

it needs substance for nourishment

Sixth unit of meaning

Basic statement

不	能	单	靠
bù	néng	dān	kào

is is not possible to solely rely on (something)

on what?

安	神 ...
ān	shén ...

on (pills) pacifying the spirit, ...

when?

在	治疗	时候
zài	zhìliáo	**shíhòu**

whenever treating (something)

160

what?

神	病
shén	bìng

spirit illnesses

Adjunct statement

必须	结合		方法	了
bìxū	jiéhé		fāngfǎ	le

it is essential to combine (them) with methods

with which methods?

养	血,	补	气	等
yǎng	xuè,	bǔ	qì	děng

(those) to nourish blood, and to supplement qi

161

Text 5.7

Sentence structures

<u>First unit of meaning</u>

Basic statement

津	和	液	是	两	种	液质
jīn	hé	yè	shì	liǎng	zhǒng	yèzhì

jin and ye are two kinds of liquids

of what kind?

不	同	性质	的
bù	tóng	xìngzhì	**de**

of dis-similar nature

Adjunct statement

但	不	等于	水	分
dàn	bù	děngyú	shuǐ	fēn

but they are not equal to watery components

which?

所	说的
suǒ	shuōde

those that are so-called (ones)

when?

一般
yībān

generally

<u>Second unit of meaning</u>

Statement

故	津液	亡脱
gù	jīnyè	wángtuō

hence when the humors are lost

162

what will happen?

为	腠理	开
wéi	còulǐ	kāi

a.)   (this) causes the pores to open

汗	大	泄
hàn	dà	**xiè**

b.)   sweat **flows off** massively

when?

在	津
zài	jīn

in case of jin (humors)

为	身体	萎枯
wéi	shēntǐ	wěikū

c.)   this causes the body to dry up

毛发	憔悴,	耳	鸣, ...
máofǎ	qiáocuì,	ěr	míng, ...

d.)   the hairs wither, the ears have sounds, ...

骨	属	屈	伸	不利
gǔ	shǔ	qū	shēn	bù lì

e.)   the bones and joints bend/stretch not freely

when?

在	液
zài	yè

in case of ye (humors)

163

<u>Third unit of meaning</u>

Basic statement

津液　可以　转化
jīnyè　kěyǐ　zhuǎnhuà

the humors can　transform

to what?

为　血
wéi　xuè

into blood

1. Adjunct statement

因而　中　　医　　有　　说法
yīn'ér zhōng　yī　　yǒu　shuōfǎ

hence Chinese medicine has an opinion

that is?

津　　　　血　　　同　　源
jīn　　　　xuè　　　tóng　yuán

jīn humors and blood have a common source

2. Adjunct statement

理由　是
lǐyóu　shì

the reason is　(as follows)

which?

亡血　有四 大　症
wángxuè yǒu sì　dà　zhèng

a.)

blood loss has four major pathoconditions

namely?

吐,　　衄,　　便,　溺
tù,　　nù,　　biàn, niào

vomiting, bleeding, stool, urine

b.)

structure identical with a.)

164

Fourth unit of meaning

Basic statement

吐	血	出	于	贲门
tù	xuè	chū	yú	bēnmén

if someone spits forth blood, it leaves from the cardia

1. Adjunct statement

与	呕吐	同
yǔ	ǒutù	tóng

that is with vomiting alike

2. Adjunct statement

鼻	衄	名	为	红	汗
bí	nù	míng	wéi	hóng	hàn

nose bleeding is termed as red sweat

3. Adjunct statement

与	汗	出	同
yǔ	hàn	chū	tóng

that is with sweat leaving (the body) alike

4. Adjunct statement: structure identical with Basic statement
5. Adjunct statement: structure identical with 1. Adjunct statement
6. Adjunct statement: structure identical with Basic statement
7. Adjunct statement: structure identical with 1. Adjunct statement

Fifth unit of meaning

Statement

两者	相比
liǎngzhě	xiāngbǐ

the two   are compared

what is the result?

性质	相似
xìngzhì	**xiāngsì**

their natures **resemble each other**

Sixth unit of meaning

Basic statement

保	津	即 所以	保	血
bǎo	jīn	jí suǒyǐ	bǎo	xuè

to protect the jin humors is, hence, to protect the blood

1. Adjunct statement

养	血	亦 可以	生	津
yǎng	xuè	yì kěyǐ	shēng	jīn

nourishing blood, too, can generate jin

2. Adjunct statement

并	提
bìng	**tí**

(we) **refer to** (something) simultaneously

to what?

亡	血	和	亡	津
wáng	xuè	hé	wáng	jīn

to losing blood and to losing jin humor

when?

常
cháng

often

where?

临症	上
línzhèng	**shàng**

in clinical practice

166

Text 5.8

Sentence structures

<u>First unit of meaning</u>

Basic statement

津　　液能化
jīn　　yè néng huà

jin and ye can transform

into what?

为 汗，　涕，　泪，涎，　　唾
wéi hàn,　tì,　　lèi, xián,　　tuò

into sweat, snivel, tears, saliva, and spittle

1. Adjunct statement

主要　　　属 于　　肾脏
zhǔyào　　shǔ yú　　shènzàng

basically they belong to　the kidneys

2. Adjunct statement

故　　称
gù　　chēng

hence it is said

what is said?

肾　主　五 液
shèn　zhǔ　wǔ yè

the kidneys rule the five ye humors

<u>Second unit of meaning</u>

Basic statement

津液　不 化
jīnyè　bù huà

the humors do not transform

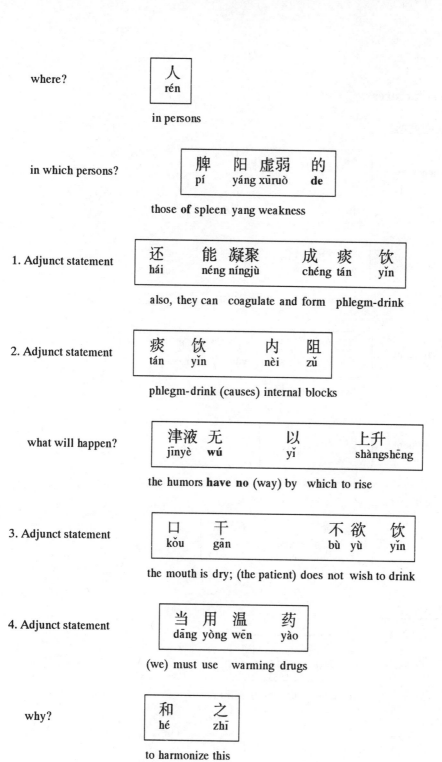

where?

人
rén

in persons

in which persons?

脾　阳　虚弱　的
pí　yáng xūruò　de

those **of** spleen yang weakness

1. Adjunct statement

还　　能 凝聚　　成 痰　饮
hái　néng níngjù　chéng tán　yǐn

also, they can coagulate and form phlegm-drink

2. Adjunct statement

痰　饮　　内　阻
tán　yǐn　nèi　zǔ

phlegm-drink (causes) internal blocks

what will happen?

津液 无　　以　　上升
jīnyè **wú**　yǐ　shàngshēng

the humors **have no** (way) by which to rise

3. Adjunct statement

口　干　　不 欲 饮
kǒu　gān　bù yù yǐn

the mouth is dry; (the patient) does not wish to drink

4. Adjunct statement

当 用 温　药
dāng yòng wēn　yào

(we) must use warming drugs

why?

和　之
hé　zhī

to harmonize this

Third unit of meaning

Basic statement

症 状　　为 口渴
zhèng zhuàng　　wéi kǒukě

one patho- manifestation is　thirst

of what kind is it?

常　　见的
cháng　　jiànde

a regularly seen (one)

where?

临症　　上
línzhèng　　**shàng**

in clinical practice

when?

津液 缺少
jīnyè quēshǎo

in case of humor deficiency

1. Adjunct statement

多　　由 热 性 病　　引起
duō　　yóu rè　xìng bìng　　**yǐnqǐ**

often it is **caused** by　heat type illnesses

2. Adjunct statement

药 为　　石斛, ... 一类
yào wéi　　shíhú, ... **yīlèi**

drugs are, **for instance**, shi-hu, ...

of which type are they?

常　　用的
cháng　　yòngde

a.)　　　　they are regularly used (ones)

169

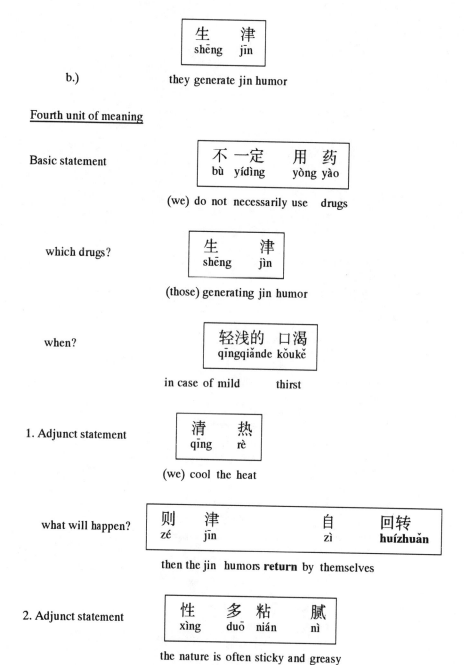

生	津
shēng	jīn

b.)   they generate jin humor

Fourth unit of meaning

Basic statement

不 一定	用 药
bù yídìng	yòng yào

(we) do not necessarily use drugs

which drugs?

生	津
shēng	jìn

(those) generating jin humor

when?

轻浅的	口渴
qīngqiǎnde	kǒukě

in case of mild   thirst

1. Adjunct statement

清	热
qīng	rè

(we) cool the heat

what will happen?

则	津	自	回转
zé	jīn	zì	**huízhuǎn**

then the jin humors **return** by themselves

2. Adjunct statement

性	多	粘	腻
xìng	duō	nián	nì

the nature is often sticky and greasy

what nature?

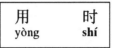

生	津	药
shēng	jīn	**yào**

(that of) **drugs** generating jin humor

3. Adjunct statement

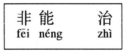

应	考虑	有无	流弊
yīng	kǎolǜ	yǒuwú	líubì

it is appropriate to consider whether it is an abuse

when?

用	时
yòng	**shí**

at the time of using (them)

Fifth unit of meaning

Basic statement

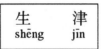

非	能	治
fēi	néng	zhì

it is not possible to cure

by doing what?

生	津
shēng	jīn

by generating jin humor

when?

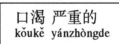

口渴	严重的
kǒukě	yánzhòngde

in cases of thirst   being severe

Adjunct statement

当	进一步	与	同	用
dāng	jìnyībù	yǔ	tóng	yòng

it is necessary to proceed   to   a simultaneous use

171

use of what?

养	血	养	阴
yǎng	xuè,	yǎng	yīn

(of drugs) to nourish blood and to nourish yin

LESSON 6: THE EXTERNAL CAUSES OF ILLNESSES

Text 6.1

Sentence structures

<u>First unit of meaning</u>

Basic statement

病　因　是　因素
bìng　yīn　shì　yīnsù

illness causes are factors

of what kind?

致　　病
zhì　　bìng

(those) leading to illness

Adjunct statement

分　　为 三　种
fēn　　wéi sān　zhǒng

(we) distinguish them into three types

namely?

内　因,　外　因, ...
nèi　yīn,　wài　yīn, ...

internal causes, external causes, ...

<u>Second unit of meaning</u>

Basic statement

以　六淫　为主
yǐ　lìu yín　wéi zhǔ

(we) hold the six excesses to be primary

in what regard?

外　因 方面
wài　yīn fāngmiàn

regarding the external causes

Adjunct statement

即 风, 寒, 署, ...
jì fēng, hán, shǔ, ...

these are wind, cold, summerheat, ...

Third unit of meaning

Basic statement

寒, ... 风 为 常 气
hán, ... fēng wéi cháng qì

cold, ... and wind are the regular qi

which regular qi?

一 年 四 季 的
yī nián sì jì **de**

(those) **of** one year's four seasons

Adjunct statement

称 为 五 气
chēng wéi wǔ qì

they are designated as the five qi

when?

在 正常的 情况 下
zài zhèngchángde qíngkuàng **xià**

under normal circumstances

Fourth unit of meaning

Basic statement

因 暑 是 热
yīn shǔ shì rè

a.) because summerheat is heat

热 极 化 火
rè jí huà huǒ

b.) (because) heat, if extreme, transforms into fire

174

	其余	亦 能 化	火
	qíyú	yì néng huà	huǒ

c.)   (because) the remaining, too, can   transform into fire

which remaining?

风,	湿,	燥,	寒
fēng,	shī,	zào,	hán

wind, dampness, dryness, and cold

when?

在	一定 条件	下
zài	yīdìng tiáojiàn	**xià**

under certain conditions

so what?

因而 将 "火"	加入
yīn'ér jiāng "huǒ"	**jiārù**

hence   fire is added

Adjunct statement

称	做	"六 气"
chēng	zuò	"liù qì"

they are designated as   the "six qi"

Fifth unit of meaning

Basic statement

六气为	正常	气 候
liù qì wéi	zhèngcháng qì	hòu

the six qi are the regular   qi manifestations

1. Adjunct statement

亦 称	"正 气"
yì chēng	"zhèng qì"

they are also called "proper qi"

175

2. Adjunct statement

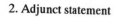

如果	非	其	时	而	有	其	气
rúguǒ	**fēi**	qí	shí	ér	**yǒu**	qí	qì

if   it **is not** its   time and yet **there is** its   qi

what is then?

便		是	反常	气	候
biàn		shì	fǎncháng	qì	hòu

then (this qi) is   an irregular qi   manifestation

3. Adjunct statement

叫	"邪 气"
jiào	"xíe qì"

it is called "evil qi"

for example?

如	风	邪,	暑	邪,	之类
rú	fēng	xié,	shǔ	xié, ...	**zhī lèi**

e.g., wind evil, heat evil, ...

4. Adjunct statement

因	这种	现象	越出	常	轨
yīn	zhèzhǒng	xiànxiàng	yuèchū	cháng	guǐ

because these   phenomena leave   the normal course

what is the result?

故	叫	"六 淫"
gù	jiào	"liù yín"

hence they are called the "six excesses"

Text 6.2

Sentence structures

<u>First unit of meaning</u>

Basic statement

风	性	多	动		善	变
fēng	**xìng**	duō	dòng		shàn	biàn

the nature of wind   is frequent movement; it tends to change

1. Adjunct statement

流行	最	广
liúxíng	zùi	guǎng

(the wind) passes over very wide (regions)

2. Adjunct statement

有	异
yǒu	yì

there are differences

which differences?

风	温,	风	热,	风	寒	之
fēng	wēn,	fēng	rè,	fēng	hán	zhī

(those) **of** wind-warmth, wind-heat, wind-cold

why?

因	季节	不	同
yīn	jìjié	bù	tóng

a.)   because the seasons are not identical

跟着	气候	转化
gēnzhe	qìhòu	zhuǎnhuà

b.)   following climatic changes

Second unit of meaning

Basic statement

(风) 结合
(fēng) jiéhé

(the wind) joins

with what?

与 其它 邪 气
yǔ qítā xié qì

with the other evil qi

to form what?

为 风 暑, 风 湿, ... 等
wéi fēng shǔ, fēng shī, ... děng

to form wind-summerheat, wind-dampness, ...

Adjunct statement

故 前 人 称 风 为 长
gù qián rén chēng fēng wéi zhǎng

hence earlier people designated the wind as chief (cause)

as chief (cause)
of what?

百 病 之
bǎi bìng **zhī**

of hundreds of illnesses

Third unit of meaning

Basic statement

感染 风 邪 发 病
gǎnrǎn fēng xié **fā** bìng

affection by wind evil **brings forth** illness

1. Adjunct statement

轻者 为 伤 风
qīngzhě wéi shāng fēng

minor ones are a "harm- caused-by-wind"

178

| where? | 在 气 分 |
| | zài qì fēn |

in the qi section

| in which qi section? | 上 焦 |
| | shàng jiāo |

(in that) of the upper burner

| 2. Adjunct statement | 出现 恶 风, ... 咳嗽 |
| | chūxiàn wù fēng, ... késou |

they produce aversion to wind, ... and cough

Fourth unit of meaning

| Basic statement | 重者 为 "中 风" |
| | zhòngzhě wéi "zhòng fēng" |

serious ones are "struck-by-wind"

| where? | 在 经 络 脏 腑 |
| | zài jīng luò zàng fǔ |

in the conduit/network (vessels), depots and palaces

| 1. Adjunct statement | 出现 口 眼 歪斜, ... |
| | chūxiàn kǒu yǎn wāixié, ... |

they produce mouth and eye wryness, ...

| 2. Adjunct statement | 轻微的 能 苏醒 |
| | qīngwēide néng sūxǐng |

mild (cases) can **regain consciousness**

179

when?

移	时
yí	shí

in the course of time

3. Adjunct statement

严重的	不 省	人	事
yánzhòngde	bù xǐng	rén	shì

serious (cases) do not recognize persons and items

Text 6.3

Sentence structures

<u>First unit of meaning</u>

Basic statement

寒 为 阴 邪
hán wéi yīn xié

cold is a yin evil

Adjunct statement

性 主 收引
xìng zhǔ **shōuyǐn**

(its) nature rules **drawing together**

<u>Second unit of meaning</u>

Basic statement

伤者 为 伤 寒
shāngzhě wéi shāng hán

harm is harmed-by-cold

harm where?

于 体 表
yú tǐ biǎo

(harm) in the body's outside

Adjunct statement

呈现 症 状
chéngxiàn zhèng zhuàng

it produces patho-manifestations

which?

恶 寒, 发热, 头痛
wù hán, fārè, tóutòng

a.)   aversion to cold, fever, headache

181

b.) the body   aches

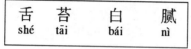

c.) the pulse appears floating and tight

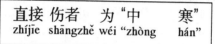

d.) the tongue coating is white and oily

Third unit of meaning

Basic statement

直接 伤者　为"中　　寒"
zhíjiē shāngzhě wéi "zhòng　hán"

direct harm   is   "struck-by-cold"

direct harm
where?

于　里
yú   lǐ

in the interior

1. Adjunct statement

呈现
chéngxiàn

it produces   (the following conditions)

namely?

呕吐 清 水
ǒutù   qīng shǔi

a.) (the patient) vomits clear liquid

182

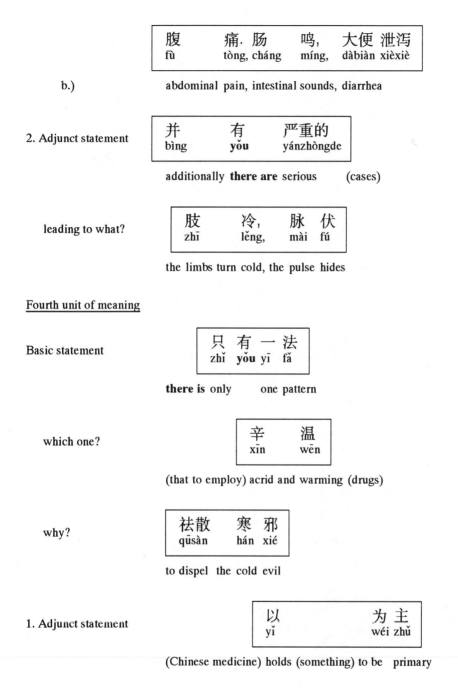

腹	痛.肠	鸣,	大便 泄泻
fù	tòng, cháng	míng,	dàbiàn xièxiè

b.)   abdominal pain, intestinal sounds, diarrhea

2. Adjunct statement

并	有	严重的
bìng	**yǒu**	yánzhòngde

additionally **there are** serious   (cases)

leading to what?

肢	冷,	脉 伏
zhī	lěng,	mài fú

the limbs turn cold, the pulse hides

Fourth unit of meaning

Basic statement

只 有 一 法
zhǐ yǒu yī fǎ

there is only   one pattern

which one?

辛	温
xīn	wēn

(that to employ) acrid and warming (drugs)

why?

祛散	寒 邪
qūsàn	hán xié

to dispel the cold evil

1. Adjunct statement

以	为主
yǐ	wéi zhǔ

(Chinese medicine) holds (something) to be primary

183

what?	解　表 jiě　biǎo

to open the outside

when?	但　　伤　　寒 dàn　　shāng　　hán

only in case of harm-caused-by-cold

2. Adjunct statement	中　寒 zhòng　hán

someone is struck by cold

what is the consequence?	则　宜　温　回 zé　yí　wēn　húi

then it is appropriate to warm and to make return

to warm what?	中 zhōng

the center

to make return what?	阳 yáng

the yang (qi)

Fifth unit of meaning

Basic statement	伤　　寒 可以 shāng　　hán kěyǐ

harm-caused-by-cold can　(do something)

184

what?

化	热
huà	rè

it transforms into heat

when?

传	变
chuán	biàn

(during) transmission and change

1. Adjunct statement

不 能	固	执
bù néng	gù	zhí

it is not possible to stubbornly cling (to something)

to what?

温	散
wēn	sàn

to warming and dispersing (therapies)

2. Adjunct statement

中	寒	少	化	热
zhòng	hán	shǎo	huà	rè

a struck-by-cold rarely transforms into heat

3. Adjunct statement

常	使	阳 气	衰退
cháng	shǐ	yáng qì	shuāituì

often it causes the yang qi to weaken

how does it
weaken?

日	渐
rì	jiàn

daily gradually

185

Text 6.4

Sentence structures

<u>First unit of meaning</u>

Statement

暑	是	主	气
shǔ	shì	zhǔ	qì

summerheat is   the ruling qi

what ruling qi?

夏令	的
xiàlìng	**de**

(that) **of** summertime

<u>Second unit of meaning</u>

Basic statement

暑	病	是 热 病
shǔ	bìng	shì rè bìng

summerheat illnesses are heat illnesses

Adjunct statement

是	分别
shì	fēnbié

(that) is   a distinction

what kind of a
distinction?

季节	上的
jìjié	**shàngde**

one **concerning** the seasons

<u>Third unit of meaning</u>

Basic statement

故	感受	暑	热
gù	gǎnshòu	shǔ	rè

hence, if (someone) was affected by summerheat-heat

186

what will happen?	多　见　热　症 duō　jiàn rè　zhèng

then (we) often see heat pathoconditions

namely?	壮　　热，口渴 心　烦，　　　自　　　汗 zhuàng rè，kǒukě xīn fán，　　　zì　　　hàn

strong heat, thirst, heart vexation, and spontaneous sweating

Adjunct statement	常　兼　　　见 喘喝，... cháng jiān　　　jiàn chuǎnhē, ...

often, jointly, (we) see panting, ...

why? a.)	由于　暑　　　热 伤　　气 yóuyú shǔ　　rè shāng　qì

because summerheat- heat harms the qi

	影响　　　心脏 yǐngxiǎng　xīnzàng

b.)   (because) it influences the heart

Fourth unit of meaning

Basic statement	暑　　热 伤　表 shǔ　rè shāng biǎo

summerheat-heat harms the outside

how?	挟　　　风 xié　　fēng

together with wind

187

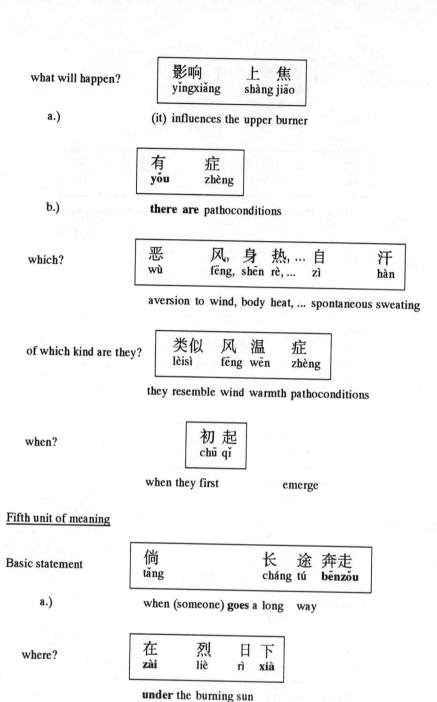

what will happen?

影响　　上焦
yǐngxiǎng　shàngjiāo

a.)　　(it) influences the upper burner

有　症
yǒu　zhèng

b.)　　**there are** pathoconditions

which?

恶　风，身　热，… 自　　汗
wù　fēng, shēn rè, … zì　hàn

aversion to wind, body heat, … spontaneous sweating

of which kind are they?

类似　风温　症
lèisì　fēng wēn　zhèng

they resemble wind warmth pathoconditions

when?

初起
chū qǐ

when they first　　　emerge

Fifth unit of meaning

Basic statement

倘　　　长途奔走
tǎng　　cháng tú bēnzǒu

a.)　　when (someone) **goes** a long　way

where?

在　烈　日　下
zài　liè　rì　xià

under the burning sun

188

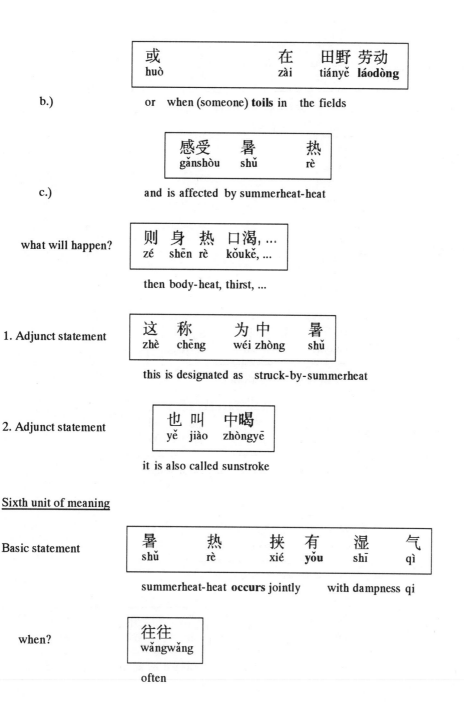

或			在	田野	劳动
huò			zài	tiányě	**láodòng**

b.)   or when (someone) **toils** in the fields

感受	暑	热
gǎnshòu	shǔ	rè

c.)   and is affected by summerheat-heat

则	身	热	口渴, ...
zé	shēn	rè	kǒukě, ...

what will happen?

then body-heat, thirst, ...

这	称	为	中	暑
zhè	chēng	wéi	zhòng	shǔ

1. Adjunct statement

this is designated as struck-by-summerheat

也	叫	中暍
yě	jiào	zhòngyē

2. Adjunct statement

it is also called sunstroke

Sixth unit of meaning

暑	热	挟	有	湿	气
shǔ	rè	xié	**yǒu**	shī	qì

Basic statement

summerheat-heat **occurs** jointly with dampness qi

往往
wǎngwǎng

when?

often

189

1. Adjunct statement

这 是　　积　　湿
zhè shì　　jī　　shī

that is: there accumulates dampness

when?

先
xiān

first

where?

内
nèi

internally

why?

由于　　郁　蒸　　的 结果
yóuyú　　yù　zhēng　**de jiéguǒ**

a.)   **because** <u>of</u> heavy steaming

why does the steaming occur?

天　　热　　地　　湿
tiān　　rè　　dì　　shī

when heaven is hot and the earth is damp

或　　　　啖 瓜果
huò　　　　dàn guāguǒ

b.)   or (someone) eats gourds

2. Adjunct statement

再　　　　　　感　暑　邪
zài　　　　　　gǎn shǔ xié

additionally, (someone) was affected by summerheat evil

190

what will happen?

则	暑	湿	愈	盛
zé	shǔ	shī	yù	shèng

then summerheat-dampness is **even more** abundant

Text 6.5

Sentence structures

<u>First unit of meaning</u>

Basic statement

湿	为	邪
shī	wéi	xié

dampness is   an evil

which evil?

重	浊	之
zhòng	zhuó	**zhī**

(that) **of** heaviness and turbidity

Adjunct statement

粘	滞
nián	zhì

a.)   it is sticky and sluggish

难	化
nán	huà

b.)   it has difficulties to transform

<u>Second unit of meaning</u>

Basic statement

多	指	潮湿
duō	zhǐ	cháoshī

often it refers to moisture

which moisture?

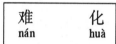

雾	露	或	天雨
wù	lù	huò	tiānyǔ

(that) of fog and dew or   rain

in which regard?	在 外 因 中
	zài wài yīn zhōng

among the external causes

Adjunct statement	感受者 发为 寒 热, …
	gǎnshòuzhě fāwéi hán rè, …

those affected develop cold and heat, …

Third unit of meaning

Basic statement	也 有
	yě yǒu

it also happens

what?	湿 邪 流 入 肌肉, 经…
	shī xié liú rù jīròu, jìng …

dampness evil flows into the flesh, the conduits …

from where?	由 皮肤
	yóu pífū

from the skin

why?	因
	yīn

because of (the following)

	坐 卧 湿 地
	zuò wò shī dì

a.)	(someone) sits or lies in a damp place

193

居处	潮湿
jūchù	cháoshī

b.)   (someone) lives   in a moist (environment)

或	水 中 作业
huò	shuǐ **zhōng** zuòyè

c.)   or (someone) <u>works</u> **in** water

汗	出	沾	衣
hàn	chū	zhān	yī

d.)   sweat flows and wets the clothes

what will happen?

则	发生	症
zé	fāshēng	zhèng

then (this) develops pathoconditions

which?

浮肿	和	关节	疼痛	等
fúzhǒng	hé	guānjié	téngtòng	děng

swelling and joint   pain

Fourth unit of meaning

Basic statement

嗜	食膏粱, ...
shì	shí gāoliáng, ...

a.)   a desire to eat rich food, ...

或 过 食	生 冷 瓜	果, ...
huò guō shí	shēng lěng guā	guǒ, ...

b.)   or   overconsumption of raw/ cold gourds and fruits, ...

194

| what will happen? | 能 使 |
| | néng shǐ |

(this) can   cause (the following)

| what? | 脾 阳   不运 |
| | pí yáng   bù yùn |

a.)   the spleen yang (qi) does not move

| | 湿   生 |
| | shī   shēng |

b.)   dampness emerges

| from where? | 自 内 |
| | zì nèi |

from the interior

| Adjunct statement | 称做 内   湿 |
| | chēngzuò nèi   shī |

(this) is called   internal dampness

Fifth unit of meaning

| Basic statement | 内 湿 在   上 |
| | nèi shī zài   shàng |

internal dampness is situated in the upper (region)

| what will happen? | 则 为 胸 闷, ... |
| | zé wéi xiōng mèn, ... |

a.)   then (this) causes chest pressure, ...

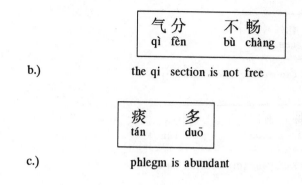

気 分　　不 畅
qì fèn　　bù chàng

b.)　　　　　　the qi section is not free

痰　　多
tán　　duō

c.)　　　　　　phlegm is abundant

1. and 2. Adjunct statement: structure identical with Basic statement

3. Adjunct statement

能 上 至 头
néng shàng zhì tóu

it can ascend to the head

what does it
cause there?

为　　面 浮
wéi　　miàn fú

it causes the face to bloat

4. Adjunct statement: structure identical with 3. Adjunct statement

196

Text 6.6

Sentence structures

<u>First unit of meaning</u>

Basic statement

燥	为	主	气
zào	wéi	zhǔ	qì

dryness is   the ruling qi

which ruling qi?

秋季
qiūjì

(that) of autumn

Adjunct statement

亦	称	秋	燥
yì	chēng	qiū	zào

it is also called autumn   dryness

<u>Second unit of meaning</u>

Basic statement

邪	多	在	上	焦
xié	duō	zài	shàng	jiāo

the evil is often situated in the upper burner

which evil?

秋	燥	之
qiū	zào	**zhī**

(that) **of** autumn dryness

how did it enter?

外	感
wài	gǎn

through external affection

197

1. Adjunct statement

类似 伤 风
lèisì shāng fēng

it resembles harm- caused- by-wind

2. Adjunct statement

表现 为 微 寒 微 热, ...
biǎoxiàn wéi wēi hán wēi rè, ...

it manifests itself as mild cold, mild heat, ...

and furthermore?

或 痰 少 粘 滞 挟 血
huò tán shǎo nián zhì xié xuè

a.)

or the phlegm is little, sticky, viscous, with blood

大便 燥 结 等
dàbiàn zào jié děng

b.)

and the stool is dry and cloddy

Third unit of meaning

Basic statement

燥 亦 为 余 气
zào yì wéi yú qì

dryness, also, is a residual qi

of what?

火 之
huǒ zhǐ

of fire

Adjunct statement

往往 发现 干燥 现象
wǎngwǎng fāxiàn gānzào xiànxiàng

there often appear dryness-signs

198

when?	热 病 之后
	rè bìng **zhīhòu**

after heat- illnesses

Fourth unit of meaning

Basic statement	燥 有 密切 关系
	zào yǒu mìqiè guānxì

dryness has a close relationship

with what?	与 津 血
	yǔ jīn xuè

with the jin humor and with blood

Adjunct statement	津 血 内 亏
	jīn xuè nèi kuī

if jin humor and blood vanish internally

what will happen?	燥 症 起
	zào zhèng qǐ

dryness pathoconditions emerge

how?	易
	yì

easily

Fifth unit of meaning

Basic statement	凡 此 皆 属 内 伤
	fán cǐ **jiē** shǔ nèi shāng

all these belong to internal harm

199

1. Adjunct statement

不 同 外 乘
bù tóng wài chéng

they are not like the external affections

affections by what?

时 气
shí qì

by the seasonal qi

which seasonal qi?

秋 燥
qiū zào

(that) of autumn dryness

2. Adjunct statement

故 当 佐入微 辛
gù dāng zuǒrù wēi xīn

hence it is essential to enter slightly acrid (drugs)

enter where?

于 甘 凉 剂 中
yú gān liáng jì zhōng

into the sweet and cooling prescriptions

when?

秋 燥
qiū zào

(in case of) autumn dryness

and for what reason?

清 泄
qīng xiè

in order to cool and to drain

3. Adjunct statement

此 则 但 宜 甘 凉
cǐ zé dàn yí gān liáng

here then however, (we) should (use) sweet and cooling (drugs)

200

why?

$$\boxed{\begin{array}{cc} 清 & 润 \\ \text{qīng} & \text{rùn} \end{array}}$$

in order to cool and to moisten

Sixth unit of meaning

Basic statement

$$\boxed{\begin{array}{ccc} 范围 & 较 & 广 \\ \text{fànwéi} & \text{jiào} & \text{guǎng} \end{array}}$$

the spectrum is relatively broad

which spectrum?

$$\boxed{\begin{array}{cc} 燥 & 症 \\ \text{zào} & \text{zhèng} \end{array}}$$

(that) of dryness pathoconditions

which dryness-
pathoconditions

$$\boxed{\begin{array}{cc} 内 & 伤 \\ \text{nèi} & \text{shāng} \end{array}}$$

(those) of inner harm

1. Adjunct statement

$$\boxed{\begin{array}{ccc} 皮肤 & 干 & 糙, \dots \\ \text{pífū} & \text{gān} & \text{cāo,} \dots \end{array}}$$

the skin   is dry and coarse, ...

where?

$$\boxed{\begin{array}{cc} 在 & 外 \\ \text{zài} & \text{wài} \end{array}}$$

in   the exterior

2. Adjunct statement: structure identical with 1. Adjunct statement

Text 6.7

Sentence structures

<u>First unit of meaning</u>

Basic statement

火	是	一	种	热	邪
huǒ	shì	yī	zhǒng	rè	xié

fire is   one type   of heat evil

in what regard?

从		外	因	方面	来说
cóng		wài	yīn	**fāngmiàn lái**	<u>shuō</u>

<u>speaking</u> **in regard of the** external causes

Adjunct statement

(火 是)	所		化
(huǒ shì)	**suǒ**		huà

(fire is)   **something that** was transformed

out of what?

由	五	气
yóu	wǔ	qì

out of the five qi

these are which?

风,	寒,	暑,	燥,	湿
fēng,	hán,	shǔ,	zào,	shī

wind, cold, summerheat, dryness, and dampness

<u>Second unit of meaning</u>

Basic statement

及	其	燔灼
jí	qí	fánzhuó

when it comes to its burning

what will happen?

则	充斥	三	焦
zé	chōngchì	sān	jiāo

then it fills　　the triple burner

1. Adjunct statement

表现
biǎoxiàn

it manifests itself (as follows)

为	口	臭,	喉	痛	红	肿
wéi	kǒu	chòu,	hóu	tòng	hóng	zhǒng

a.)　　as　mouth odor, throat pain, redness, swelling

胸	闷	烦躁
xiōng	mèn	fánzào

b.)　　chest pressure and vexation

腹	满	溲	赤
fù	mǎn	sǒu	chì

c.)　　abdominal fullness and urine redness

2. Adjunct statement

甚	至
shèn	zhì

in severe cases it comes (to the following conditions)

发	斑	发	疹
fā	bān	fā	zhěn

a.)　　it develops macules and it develops papules

203

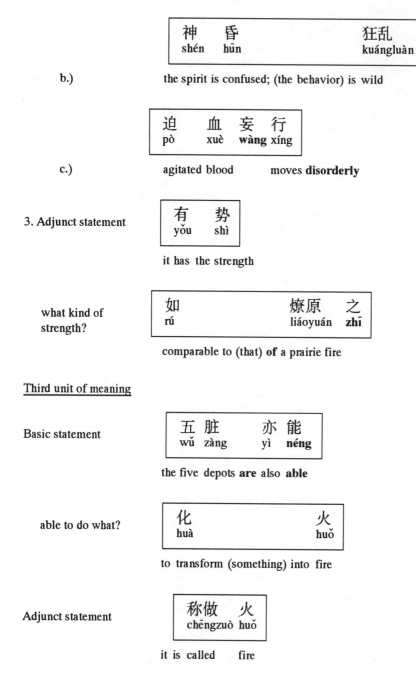

神　昏　　　　　　　狂乱
shén　hūn　　　　　　kuángluàn

b.)　　　　　the spirit is confused; (the behavior) is wild

迫　血　妄　行
pò　xuè　**wàng** xíng

c.)　　　　　agitated blood　　moves **disorderly**

3. Adjunct statement　　有　势
yǒu　shì

it has the strength

what kind of　　如　　　　　燎原　之
strength?　　　rú　　　　　liáoyuán　**zhī**

comparable to (that) **of a prairie fire**

Third unit of meaning

Basic statement　　五　脏　亦　能
wǔ　zàng　yì　**néng**

the five depots **are** also **able**

able to do what?　　化　　　　　火
huà　　　　　huǒ

to transform (something) into fire

Adjunct statement　　称做　火
chēngzuò huǒ

it is called　　fire

204

which fire?

五	志	之
wǔ	zhì	**zhī**

(that) **of** the five emotions

Fourth unit of meaning

Basic statement

以	火	最	为	多	见
yǐ	huǒ	**zuì**	wéi	duō	jiàn

(we) consider the fire   as **most** often visible

which fire?

肝	胆	之
gān	dǎn	**zhī**

(that) **of** liver and gallbladder

Adjunct statement

症	现	目 赤, ...	等
zhèng	xiàn	mù chì, ...	děng

as pathoconditions appear eye redness, ...

Fifth unit of meaning

Basic statement

火	多	为	实	火
huǒ	duō	wéi	shí	huǒ

fire often is   repletion fire

which fire?

不论	五	气	化
bùlùn	wǔ	qì	huà

regardless whether the five qi have transformed

或	五	志	之
huò	wǔ	zhì	**zhī**

or   whether it is (a fire) **of** the five emotions

1. Adjunct statement

当		用 苦	寒
dāng		yòng kǔ	hán

it is necessary to use   bitter and cold (substances)

what for?

直	折
zhí	zhé

to directly break it

2. Adjunct statement

不 是	所		能 治疗
bù shì	suǒ		néng zhìliáo

it   is   **not** <u>that which</u> (prescriptions) can   cure

which prescriptions?

一般	清	热 剂
yībān	qīng	rè jì

those commonly cooling the heat prescriptions

Text 6.8

Sentence structures

<u>First unit of meaning</u>

Basic statement

邪　发　　　病
xié　fā　　　bìng

an evil brings forth an illness

which evil?

感染　之
gǎnrǎn　zhī

(that) **of** an affection

an affection by what?

六　淫
liù　yín

(an affection by one) of the six　excesses

when?

不　即
bù　jí

not immediately

1. Adjunct statement

出现　病症
chūxiàn　bìngzhèng

it produces illness-conditions

when?

经过 一个 相当　时期 方才
jīngguò yīgè　xiāngdāng shíqī　fāngcái

after　a　　suitable　time,　only then

2. Adjunct statement

例如,　　受了　　寒　邪
lìrú,　　shòule　hán xié

if one, e. g.,　has received a cold evil

when?

冬天
dōngtiān

in winter

what will happen?

生	温	病
shēng	wēn	bìng

then this generates a warmth illness

when?

到	夏天	才
dào	xiàtiān	cái

when it comes to summer, then

3. Adjunct statement: structure identical with 2. Adjunct statement

<u>Second unit of meaning</u>

这	称做	伏	邪
zhè	chēngzùo	fú	xíe

that is called   "hidden evil"

<u>Third unit of meaning</u>

Statement

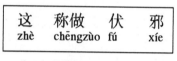

邪 为	因素 之 一
xíe wéi	yīnsù **zhī** yī

the evil is   <u>one</u> **of** the factors

which evil?

疫疠	之
yìlì	**zhī**

(that) **of** epidemics

one of which factors?

外 来	致 病
wài lái	zhì bìng

those   coming from **outside** to cause illness

Fourth unit of meaning

Basic statement

疫	是	互相	染易
yì	shì	hùxiāng	rǎnyì

"yi" is   mutual   passage

1. Adjunct statement

病	状	相	似
bìng	zhuàng	xiāng	sì

the illness manifestations are mutually alike

in what regard?

不问	大	小
bùwèn	dà	xiǎo

regardless whether adults or children (are concerned)

2. Adjunct statement

即	意思
jí	yìsī

that is   the meaning

of what?

传染	的
chuánrǎn	**de**

(that) **of** "infection"

Fifth unit of meaning

Basic statement

疠	指	一	种	气
lì	zhǐ	yī	zhǒng	qì

"li" refers to one type   of qi

to which type of qi?

毒	戾	之
dú	lì	**zhī**

(to that) **of** poison and viciousness

where?

自然界
zìránjiè

in nature

1. Adjunct statement

危害	健康	最	大
wēihài	jiànkāng	zuì	dà

it endangers health   most massively

2. Adjunct statement

不	同	于	普通的	邪
bù	tóng	yú	pǔtōngde	xié

it is not identical with the common evils

with which common evils?

六	淫	之
liù	yín	**zhī**

(with those) **of** the six excesses

Sixth unit of meaning

Basic statement

发生	(是)	所	成
fāshēng	(shì)	**suǒ**	chéng

the emergence (is)   **that which** is formed

what emergence?

疠	气	的
lì	qì	**de**

(that) **of** li   qi

210

out of what is
it formed?

由　　酝酿
yóu　　yùnniàng

out of transformation

when?

淫　　雨,　　亢　旱
yín　　yǔ,　　kàng　hàn

a.)

in case of excessive rain and severe drought

或　　　家畜　　　瘟　死
huò　　jiāchù　　wēn　sǐ

b.)

or when the livestock **died** of an epidemic

秽　物　腐败
huì　wù　fǔbài

c.)

and when filthy items decay

Seventh unit of meaning

Basic statement

分为　　两　项
fēnwéi　　liǎng xiàng

(we) distinguish two   types

which two types?

寒　疫　　和　瘟　疫
hán　yì　　hé　wēn　yì

cold epidemics and warmth epidemics

in what regard?

从　　　性质　上
cóng　　xìngzhì **shàng**

seen **from** (their) nature

211

1. Adjunct statement

吸　　受
xī　　shòu

they are inhaled and taken in

how?

由 口　　鼻
yóu kǒu　　bí

by mouth and nose

2. Adjunct statement

入　　肠　　胃
rù　　cháng　　wèi

they enter the intestines and the stomach

how?

直
zhí

directly

3. Adjunct statement

发　　病
fā　　bìng

they develop an illness

how?

极 速
jí　sù

very quickly

212

LESSON 7: THE INTERNAL CAUSES OF ILLNESS

Text 7.1

Sentence structures

<u>First unit of meaning</u>

Basic statement

以　　　七　情　为　主
yǐ　　　qī　qíng　wéi zhǔ

(we) consider the seven affects as primary

in what regard?

内　　因
nèi　　yīn

(in regard to) the internal causes

1. Adjunct statement

还　　　有　　痰,　瘀, ...　　　等
hái　　　yǒu　　tán,　yū, ...　　　děng

additionally **there are** phlegm, stagnations, ...

2. Adjunct statement

同　为　　　重要　因素
tóng wéi　　　zhòngyào yīnsù

they　　are **equally** important factors

<u>Second unit of meaning</u>

Statement

七　情　即 忧, ...　　惊
qī　qíng　jī yōu, ...　　jīng

the seven affects are sorrow, ... and fright

213

Third unit of meaning

Basic statement

病	是 一 种	情志	病
bìng	shì yī zhǒng	qíngzhì	bìng

the illnesses are one type   of emotional illness

which illnesses?

七	情	发
qī	qíng	**fā**

(those, which) the seven affects **bring forth**

Adjunct statement

是	因于
shǐ	yīnyú

that is   so because of (the following)

namely?

刺激	使	发生 变化
cìjī	shǐ	fāshēng biànhuà

a stimulus causes (a person) to develop changes

where?

精神	上
jīngshén	**shàng**

in the mind

what kind of stimulus?

外界	事物 的
wàijìe	shìwù **de**

(one) **of** an environmental entity

Fourth unit of meaning

Statement

变化 有 反映
biànhuà yǒu fǎnyìng

the changes have reflections

214

which changes?

精神 的
jīngshén **de**

(those) **of** the mind

which reflections?

不同的
bùtóngde

different (ones)

why?

由于 不 同
yóuyú bù tóng

because of dis- similarities

which dissimilarities?

外界 刺激 的
wàijiè cìjī **de**

(those) **of** the environmental stimuli

Fifth unit of meaning

Basic statement

症 状 如 抑郁 ...
zhèng zhuàng rú yìyù ...

patho- manifestations are, e.g., depression ...

which patho-
manifestations?

常 见的
cháng jiànde

often seen (ones)

1. Adjunct statement

严重的 神志 恍惚,...
yánzhòngde shēnzhì huǎnghū,...

serious (cases) are absentmindedness,...

2. Adjunct statement

如	癫	如	痴
rú	diān	rú	chī

they resemble insanity, they resemble idiocy

Sixth unit of meaning

Statement

病	变	是	变化
bìng	biàn	shì	biànhuà

pathological changes are transformations

which pathological changes?

引起的
yǐnqǐde

brought forth (ones)

brought forth by what?

七	情
qī	qíng

(by) the seven affects

transformations of what?

气	的
qì	de

(those) of qi

Seventh unit of meaning

Basic statement

影响	是	气
yǐngxiǎng	shì	qì

the influence is on the qi

what influence?

七	情	的
qī	qíng	de

(that) of the seven affects

216

when?

最　先
zuì　xiān

on the very first

1. Adjunct statement

气 与 血　是 不 可分离的
qì yǔ xuè　shì bù kěfēnlíde

qi　and blood are　not　separable

2. Adjunct statement

故　　病情　　进一步　　影响 到 血
gù　　bìngqíng　　jìnyībù　　yǐngxiǎng dào xuè

hence the illness　　has, furthermore, an influence　on　the blood

Text 7.2

Sentence structures

First unit of meaning

Basic statement

似		可	作	为 外	因
sì		kě	zuò	wéi wài	yīn

it seems as if they could be regarded as external causes

what?

变化
biànhuà

the changes

which changes?

七	情
qī	qíng

(those) of the seven affects

why?

既	引起
jì	yǐnqǐ

because they are brought forth

brought forth by what?

由 外	界	刺激
yóu wài	jiè	cìjī

by external world stimuli

Adjunct statement

但是	毕竟	不 一样
dànshì	bìjìng	bù yīyàng

however, finally this is not identical

with what?

与	外	因	发	病
yǔ	wài	yīn	fā	bìng

with how the external causes **bring forth** illnesses

218

which external causes?

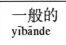
一般的
yībānde

the common (ones)

Second unit of meaning

Basic statement

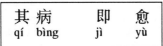
只　要　　去　其　　　外　　因
zhǐ　yào　　qù　qí　　　wài　yīn

it is only necessary to　remove their external causes

when?

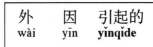
外　　　因　　引起的
wài　　yīn　　yǐnqǐde

(in case of illness) **brought forth** by external causes

what is
the result?

其　病　　　即　　愈
qí　bìng　　jì　　yù

this illness will then be cured

Adjunct statement

七　　情　　　起到　变化
qī　　qíng　　qǐdào　biànhuà

the seven affects have effected changes

when?

已经
yǐjing

already

where?

在　　精神　上
zài　jīngshén **shàng**

in　the mind

219

and furthermore?

并　　使　　改变
bìng　shǐ　gǎibiàn

also, they stimulate changes

what changes?

内在的生活　　情况
nèizàide shēnghuǒ　qíngkuàng

(those) of internal physiological conditions

what will happen?

即　　　　使　　刺激　不再　存在 时
jí　　　　shǐ　cìjī　bù zài　cúnzài shí

then, **as soon as** (we) cause the stimulus no longer to exist

也 不 能　立即　恢复
yě bù néng　lìjí　huīfù

(the patient) is still not able to immediately recover

Third unit of meaning

Statement

同样的 病　有 差别
tóngyàngde bìng　yǒu chābié

identical illnesses have differences

which identical
illnesses?

七　情
qī　qíng

(those brought forth by) the seven affects

which differences?

显著的
xiǎnzhùde

obvious　(ones)

220

in what regard?

在　　　　病　症　　　上
zài　　　bìng　zhèng　**shàng**

as regards the illness conditions

why?

由于　　　刺激　有　强　　　弱
yóuyú　　　cìjī　yǒu　qiáng　　ruò

because the stimuli have strong and weak (variants)

Fourth unit of meaning

Basic statement

体质　　　和　敏感性　　有　　关系
tǐzhì　　　hé　mǐngǎnxìng　yǒu　guānxì

constitution and susceptibility have a relationship

what constitution
and susceptibility?

病人　的
bìngrén **de**

(those) **of** the patient

what kind of a
relationship?

极　大
jí　dà

a very great (one)

relationship
to what?

对 受　　　病
duì shòu　　　bìng

to　contracting an illness

Adjunct statement

需要　仔细　观察
xūyào　zǐxì　guānchá

(we) must　carefully　examine (them)

221

Text 7.3

Sentence structures

<u>First unit of meaning</u>

Basic statement

脾　阳　　衰弱
pí　yáng　shuāiruò

the spleen yang is weak

what will happen?

a.)

水湿　　不化
shuǐshī　bù huà

liquids do not transform

b.)

凝聚　　成　痰
níngjù　chéng tán

they coagulate to form　phlegm

Adjunct statement

肺　热　煎熬　　津液
fèi　rè　jiān'áo　jīnyè

when lung heat boils　the fluids of the body

what will happen?

亦　能　成　痰
yì　néng chéng tán

that, too, can　form　phlegm

<u>Second unit of meaning</u>

Statement

以　　　　　为密切
yǐ　　　　wéi mìqiè

(we) consider (something) to be　close

222

what?

肺 和 脾
fèi hé pí

(the relationships to) lung and spleen

how close?

最
zuì

very (close)

in what regard?

关系
guānxì

(in regard to) the relationships

which relationships?

痰　　与　　内　脏　的
tán　　yú　　nèi　zàng　de

(those) **of** phlegm to   the inner depots

Third unit of meaning

Basic statement

主要　症　状　　为 咳嗽
zhǔyào zhèng zhuàng   wéi késou

the primary patho-manifestion is   cough

which primary patho-
manifestation?

痰　　　　　的
tán　　　　　de

(that) **of** phlegm (illnesses)

1. Adjunct statement

阻碍　　肃降
zǔ'ài　　sùjiàng

(phlegm) blocks the descending (movement)

which descending movement?

气 机　　　的
qì jī　　　de

(that) **of** the qi　dynamics

what will happen?

则　　　为　　　喘息
zé　　　wéi　　　chuǎnxī

then this causes panting

2. Adjunct statement

亦 能　　　流 窜
yì néng　　　liú cuàn

it is also able to flow through (something)

through what?

经　　　　络
jīng　　　　luò

the conduits and the network (vessels)

what will happen?

出现　症
chūxiàn　zhèng

(that) produces pathoconditions

which pathoconditions?

手　　　足　　　麻木, ...
shǒu　　　zú　　　mámù, ...

hands and feet being numb, ..

Fourth unit of meaning

Basic statement

若　　　　和 其它 因素 结合
ruò　　　　hé qítā yīnsù **jiéhé**

when it **merges** with other factors

224

what will happen?

有	寒 痰, ...
yǒu	hán tán, ...

a.) **there is** cold phlegm, ...

则	症 状	更	为 复杂	了
zé	zhèng zhuàng	gèng	wéi fùzá	le

b.) then the patho- manifestations **are** <u>even more</u> complex

Fifth unit of meaning

Basic statement

痰	占有	地位
tán	zhànyǒu	dìwèi

phlegm occupies a position

what kind of
a position?

重要
zhòngyào

an important (position)

where?

在	病 因	中
zài	bìng yīn	zhōng

among the illness causes

1. Adjunct statement

病症	能 引起	痰	浊
bìngzhèng	néng yǐnqǐ	tán	zhuó

illness conditions can **give rise** to phlegm turbidity

all illness
conditions?

很 多
hěn duō

very many

in what regard?

除了　　病　　之外
chúle　　bìng　　zhīwài

in addition to illnesses

which illnesses?

因　　痰　　生
yīn　　tán　　shēng

those **generated** because of phlegm

2. Adjunct statement

既　　必须　　　　兼 顾
jí　　bìxū　　　　jiān gù

hence (we) must　**consider** (this) too

when?

有 痰　浊
yǒu tán　zhuó

when (a patient) has phlegm turbidity

226

Text 7.4

Sentence structures

<u>First unit of meaning</u>

Basic statement

饮　　食　为 泉源
yǐn　　shí　wéi quányuán

drink and food are sources

sources of what?

营养　　　的
yíngyǎng　　**de**

of nourishment

Adjunct statement

但 恣贪　　口腹, 没有 节制, ...
dàn zìtān　　kǒufù, méiyǒu jiézhì, ...

but indulging in food　without restraint, ...

亦 能 致　病
yì néng zhì　bìng

they too can　lead to illness

<u>Second unit of meaning</u>

Statement

称　　　　做 伤　　　食
chēng　　　zuò shāng　　shí

(we) designate (something) as　harm caused by food

what?

痞　　闷
pǐ　　mèn

a.)　　　　blocks and pressure

where?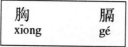

in the chest and at the diaphragm

b.: structure identical with a.

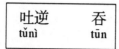

c.) vomiting and regurgitation

what ist regurgitated?

(stomach) acid

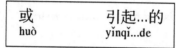

d.) or (conditions) bringing forth (something)

what do they bring forth?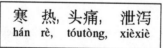

cold heat, headache, diarrhea

Third unit of meaning

Statement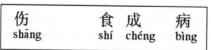

harm caused by food generates illnesses

where?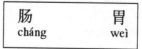

(in) the intestines and the stomach

228

when?

often

Fourth unit of meaning

Basic statement

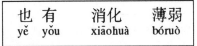

it also happens: digestion is weak

in what regard?

originally

1. Adjunct statement

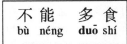

(the patient) is not able to   eat **much**

2. Adjunct statement

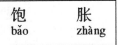

fullness and distension (result)

when?

after the meals

3. Adjunct statement

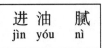

(someone) eats oily or greasy (food)

how much?

稍
shāo

little

what will happen?

大便　溏薄
dàbiàn　tángbó

the stool　is semiliquid

4. Adjunct statement

中　医　称为　脾　虚
zhōng　yī　chēngwéi　pí　xū

Chinese medicine calls　(that) spleen depletion

Fifth unit of meaning

Basic statement

以　能　食不　消化
yǐ　néng　shí bù　xiāohùa

it considers an ability to eat without digestion

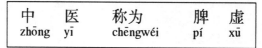

为胃　强　脾　弱
wéi wèi　qiáng　pí　ruò

as　stomach strength and spleen　weakness

Adjunct statement: structure identical with Basic statement

Text 7.5

Sentence structures

<u>First unit of meaning</u>

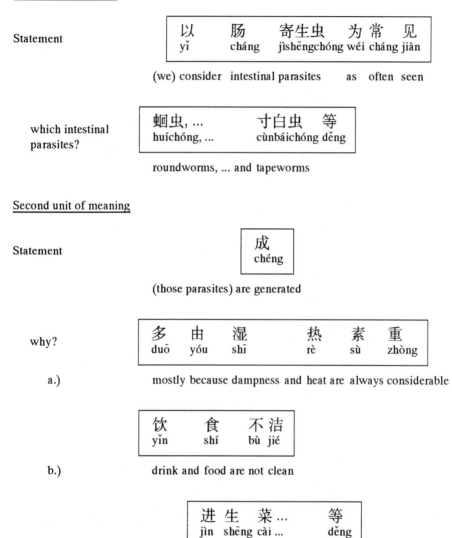

Statement

以	肠	寄生虫	为 常 见
yǐ	cháng	jìshēngchóng	wéi cháng jiàn

(we) consider intestinal parasites   as   often seen

which intestinal
parasites?

蛔虫, ...	寸白虫 等
huíchóng, ...	cùnbáichóng děng

roundworms, ... and tapeworms

<u>Second unit of meaning</u>

Statement

成
chéng

(those parasites) are generated

why?

多	由	湿	热	素	重
duō	yóu	shī	rè	sù	zhòng

a.)   mostly because dampness and heat are always considerable

饮	食	不洁
yǐn	shí	bù jié

b.)   drink and food are not clean

进 生 菜 ...	等
jìn shēng cài ...	děng

c.)   someone eats raw   vegetables, ...

how?

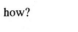

mixed

Third unit of meaning

Basic statement

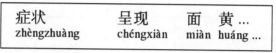

症状　　　　呈现　　　面　黄...
zhèngzhuàng　chéngxiàn　miàn　huáng...

the pathomanifestations appear　as facial yellowness ...

which
pathomanifestations?

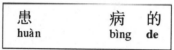

患　　　　病　的
huàn　　　bìng　de

(those) of suffering from an illness

from which illness?

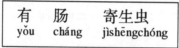

有　肠　　寄生虫
yǒu　cháng　jìshēngchóng

that of having intestinal parasites

1. Adjunct statement

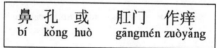

鼻　孔　或　肛门　作痒
bí　kǒng　huò　gāngmén　zuòyǎng

the nose holes or　the anus　itches

2. Adjunct statement

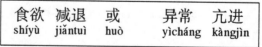

唇　内　生　白　点　如　　粟　粒
chún nèi　shēng　bái　diǎn rú　　sù　lì

the lip　interior develops white dots resembling millet grains

3. Adjunct statement

食欲　减退　或　　异常　亢进
shíyù　jiǎntuì　huò　　yìcháng　kàngjìn

the appetite decreases or　shows abnormal hyperfunction

232

4. Adjunct statement

有的嗜　　食生米，茶叶
yǒude shì　　shí shēng mǐ,　chá yè

some prefer to eat raw　rice or tea leaves

5. Adjunct statement

腹　　内　　阵痛
fù　　nèi　　zhèn tòng

the abdominal interior has labor pain

6. Adjunct statement

面部 变　　色
miànbù biàn　　sè

the face　　changes its color

Fourth unit of meaning

Basic statement

酿成　疳　　积
niàngchéng gān　　jī

(parasites) produce　malnutrition accumulation

where?

在 小 儿
zài xiǎo ér

in small children

how?

尤　　易
yóu　　yì

especially easily

1. Adjunct statement

腹　　大, 坚,　　满
fù　　dà, jiān,　　mǎn

the abdomen grows big, hardens, and is full

2. Adjunct statement

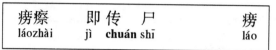

俗　　呼　疳　　膨...
sú　　hū　gān　　péng...

that is commonly called malnutrition inflation...

Fifth unit of meaning

Basic statement

痨瘵　　即传尸　　　　　痨
láozhài　　jì　**chuán** shī　　　　láo

consumption is　　　　corpse-**transmitted** consumption

1. Adjunct statement

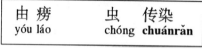

由痨　　　虫　传染
yóu láo　　chóng　**chuánrǎn**

it is **transmitted** by consumption worms

2. Adjunct statement

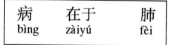

病　　在于　　肺
bìng　zàiyú　　fèi

the illness is situated in the lung

Sixth unit of meaning

Basic statement

症　　　见　咳嗽 ...
zhèng　　jiàn　késou ...

as pathoconditions appear cough, ...

Adjunct statement

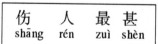

伤　人　最　甚
shāng　rén　zuì　shèn

(this illness) harms a person very severely

234

Text 7.6

Sentence structures

First unit of meaning

Statement

虽	分	外	因	和 内	因
suí	fēn	wài	yīn	hé nèi	yīn

although (we) distinguish external causes and internal causes

in what regard?

病	因
bìng	yīn

(in regard to) illness causes

but?

但	不 能	把 它们	看
dàn	bù néng	**bǎ tāmen**	kàn

but it is not possible   to view **them**

view them how?

孤立起来
gūlìqǐlái

separately

Second unit of meaning

Basic statement

中	医	分	疾病
zhōng	yī	fēn	jíbìng

Chinese medicine distinguishes the illnesses

为 两	类
wéi liǎng	lèi

into two   categories

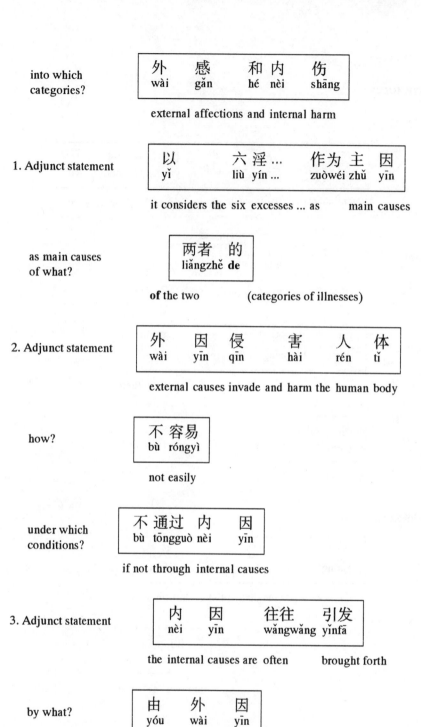

into which categories?

外　感　　和内　伤
wài　gǎn　　hé nèi　shāng

external affections and internal harm

1. Adjunct statement

以　　　六淫 ...　作为主　因
yǐ　　　liù yín ...　zuòwéi zhǔ　yīn

it considers the six excesses ... as　　main causes

as main causes of what?

两者　的
liǎngzhě **de**

of the two　　　(categories of illnesses)

2. Adjunct statement

外　因　侵　　害　　人　体
wài　yīn　qīn　　hài　　rén　tǐ

external causes invade and harm the human body

how?

不 容易
bù róngyì

not easily

under which conditions?

不 通过 内　　因
bù tōngguò nèi　　yīn

if not through internal causes

3. Adjunct statement

内　因　　往往　引发
nèi　yīn　　wǎngwǎng yǐnfā

the internal causes are often　　brought forth

by what?

由　外　因
yóu　wài　yīn

by　the external causes

how?

同样地
tóngyàngde

similarly

Third unit of meaning

Basic statement

同是		应当	注意		其它	因素
tóngshì		yīngdāng	**zhùyì**		qítā	yīnsù

similarly (we) should **pay attention to** other factors

in which
regard?

除了		主	因	之外
chúle		zhǔ	yīn	**zhīwài**

in addition to the major causes

what major
causes?

发... 的
fā... de

(those) bringing forth (something)

what?

病
bìng

the illnesses

for instance?

如	生活,	营养,		居住	条件	等
rú	shēnghuǒ	yíngyǎng		jūzhù	tiáojiàn	děng

e.g., life (style), nourishment, and housing conditions

Adjunct statement

均有	极	大	关系
jūn yǒu	jí	dà	guānxì

they all have a very great association (with illness)

Text 7.7

Sentence structures

<u>First unit of meaning</u>

Basic statement

发生	有	意外	损害
fāshēng	yǒu	yìwài	sǔnhài

an emergence has an accidental injury (as its cause)

emergence
of what?

疾病	的
jíbìng	**de**

of an illness

so what?

既不	属	于	内	因
jìbù	shǔ	yú	nèi	yīn

a.)   neither does it belong to the internal causes

又不	属	于	外	因
yòubù	shǔ	yú	wài	yīn

b.)   nor does it belong to the external causes

Adjunct statement

称	为	不	内	外	因
chēng	wéi	bù	nèi	wài	yīn

(we) designate this as "neither- internal- nor- external-cause"

<u>Second unit of meaning</u>

Statement

房室	伤	指	受伤
fángshì	shāng	zhǐ	shòushāng

bedroom-caused-harm refers to harm

harm to what?

精	气
jīng	qì

to essence and qi

caused by what?

色欲	过度
sèyù	guòdù

caused by sexual excesses

Third unit of meaning

Statement

不仅	身体	虚	弱
bù jǐn	shēntǐ	xū	ruò

not only the body is depleted and weak

but also?

还	招致	病	邪
hái	zhāozhì	bìng	xié

it also invites an illness evil

how?

易
yì

easily

Fourth unit of meaning

Statement

金刃	伤	指	一	类
jīnrèn	shāng	zhǐ	yī	lèi

weapon-caused-harm refers to one group

which group?

创伤	或	损伤
chuāngshāng	huò	sǔnshāng

(that) of wounds   or injuries

239

which kind of wounds?

刀　剑
dāo　jiàn

(those caused by) knives or swords

which kind of injuries?

跌打
diē-dǎ

(those caused by) accidental falls

Fifth unit of meaning

Statement

汤　火伤
tāng　huǒ shāng

harm (caused by) hot liquids or fire

指　烫伤　或 烧伤
zhǐ　tàngshāng huò shāoshāng

refers to scalding　or　burns

scaldings by what?

汤水
tāng shuǐ

by hot water

burns by what?

火灼
huǒzhuó

by fire

Sixth unit of meaning

Basic statement

虫 兽　　伤 指　咬伤
chóng shòu　shāng zhǐ　yǎo shāng

insect/animal-(caused)-harm refers to bite harm

240

| bite-harm caused by what? | 毒 蛇 猛 兽 |
| | dú shé měng shòu |

by poisonous snakes and wild animals

| Adjunct statement | 还 能 引起 中毒 |
| | hái néng yǐnqǐ zhòngdú |

they also can evoke poisonings

| which kind of poisonings? | 不同 程度 的 |
| | bùtóng chéngdù de |

(those) **of** different degrees

| in what regard? | 除了 直接 伤害 外 |
| | **chúle** zhíjiē shānghài **wài** |

in addition to direct wounds

| of which kind? | 体 表 受到 |
| | tǐ biǎo shòudào |

(those which) the body outside receives

Seventh unit of meaning

| Statement | 中毒 指 食物 中毒 或 ... |
| | zhòngdú zhǐ shíwù zhòngdú huò ... |

poisoning refers to food poisoning or ...

| when? | 一般 多 |
| | yībān duō |

generally, mostly

Basic statement

不	内	外	因	有	关系
bù	nèi	wài	yīn	yǒu	guānxì

the neither-internal- nor-external causes have relationships

to what?

和	内	因,		外	因
hé	nèi	yīn,		wài	yīn

to the internal causes, and to the external causes

Adjunct statement

譬如	外	邪	侵入
pìrú	wài	xié	qīnrù

e.g., an external evil invades (the body)

when?

刀	伤	后
dāo	shāng	hòu

after a knife caused harm

how does it enter?

从	创	口
cóng	chuāng	kǒu

through the wound opening

what will happen?

能	发生	破伤风症
néng	fāshēng	pòshāngfēngzhèng

it can evoke a tetanus condition

what kind of a tetanus condition?

严	重的
yán	zhòngde

a very serious (one)

Ninth unit of meaning

Statement

不 能 把 它	孤立起来
bù néng <u>bǎ</u> <u>tā</u>	gūlìqǐlái

(we)   can   **not** isolate <u>it</u>

what?

任何 一	因, 都
rènhé yī	yīn, **dōu**

each   single   cause

where?

三	因	中
sān	yīn	**zhōng**

among the three causes

Text 7.8

Sentence structures

<u>First unit of meaning</u>

Basic statement

来	必	有	因
lái	bì	yǒu	yīn

an arrival must have a cause

arrival of what?

病	之
bìng	**zhī**

of an illness

1. Adjunct statement

一个	原因	可以	生出	病
yīgè	yuányīn	kěyǐ	shēngchū	bìng

one cause can generate illnesses

what kind
of illnesses?

多	种	不	同的
duō	zhǒng	bù	tóngde

many types, dis- similar (ones)

2. Adjunct statement

同一	病症	可	造成
tóngyī	bìngzhèng	kě	zàochéng

one identical illness can be generated

by what?

由	各	种	不	同的	原因
yóu	gè	zhǒng	bù	tóngde	yuányīn

by all kinds of dis- similar causes

Second unit of meaning

Basic statement

所以	中	医	有	特点
suǒyǐ	zhōng	yī	**yǒu**	tèdiǎn

hence Chinese medicine has a characteristic

which characteristic?

异	病	同	治,
yì	bìng	tóng	zhì,

(that) **of** "different illnesses identical treatment,

同	病	异	治	的
tóng	bìng	yì	zhì	**de**

identical illnesses different treatment"

1. Adjunct statement

一个	药	方	治	病
yīgè	yào	fāng	zhì	bìng

one drug formula cures illnesses

illnesses
of what kind?

几	种	不 同的
jǐ	zhǒng	bù tóngde

several kinds of dis- similar (ones)

2. Adjunct statement

必须	用	几个	药	方
bìxū	yòng	jǐgè	yào	fāng

it is necessary to use several drug formulas

when?

有时	在	一	种	病	上
yǒushí	**zài**	yī	zhǒng	bìng	**shàng**

sometimes, **in case of** one single type of illness

245

why?	来 治疗 lái zhìliáo
	to cure (it)

Third unit of meaning

Basic statement	有的 表现 为 发热 yǒude biǎoxiàn wéi fārè
	some appear as fever

for example?	例如, 同一 热 邪 lìrú, tóngyī rè xié
	e.g., identical heat evil

1. Adjunct statement	有的 咳嗽 yǒude késòu
	some (appear as) cough

2. Adjunct statement: structure identical with 1. Adjunct statement

3. Adjunct statement	要 求得是 热 邪 yào qíudé shì rè xié
	it is necessary to find this heat evil

4. Adjunct statement	病症 虽 异 bìngzhèng suí yì
	the illness conditions may differ

but?	都 能 用 清凉 剂 dōu néng yòng qīngliáng jì
	in all cases it is possible to use cooling formulas

Fourth unit of meaning

Basic statement

如 同一　发热
rú　tóngyī　fārè

if　identical fevers (appear)

what are they?

有　　　起的
yǒu　　qǐde

there are brought forth (ones)

brought forth
because of what?

因　　　热 邪, ... 而
yīn　　rè　xié, ... **ér**

because of heat evil, ...

1. Adjunct statement

发热 虽　同
fārè　suí　tóng

the fevers　may be identical

but?

而　　原因　　不 同
ér　　yuányīn　bù tóng

but the causes　are not identical

which causes?

所以　　　　　引起...的
suǒyǐ　　　　yǐnqǐ...de

(those) by which (something) was brought forth

what?

发热
fārè

the fever

2. Adjunct statement

不 能　　专　　用
bù néng　　zhuān　　yòng

it is not possible to exclusively use　(something)

to use what?

清凉　剂
qīngliáng jì

cooling　formulas

to achieve what?

退　　热
tùi　　rè

to repel the heat

Fifth unit of meaning

Basic statement

这 是　　说明　　重要性
zhè shì　　shuōmíng　　zhòngyàoxìng

that is　to explain　the importance

what importance?

病　因　对于　　治疗 的
bìng　yīn　duìyú　　zhìliáo **de**

(that) **of** illness causes vis-a-vis a therapy

1. Adjunct statement

治疗 任何一 种　病
zhìliáo rènhéyī　zhǒng bìng

to treat　any　type of illness

what is necessary?

要　　弄清楚
yào　　nòngqīngchǔ

it is necessary to clarify　(something)

248

what?

原因
yuányīn

the causes

when?

首先
shǒuxiān

first

LESSON 8: THE EIGHT PRINCIPLES

Text 8.1

Sentence structures

<u>First unit of meaning</u>

Basic statement

每 一个 病 都 有 症状
měi yīgè bìng **dōu** yǒu zhèngzhuàng

each single illness has pathomanifestations

of what kind?

错综 复杂的
cuòzōng fùzáde

complex (ones)

Adjunct statement

要 找到 它的关键
yào zhǎodào tāde guānjiàn

(we) wish to find out its keypoints

掌握 它的主要 方面
zhǎngwò tāde zhǔyào fāngmiàn

and to grasp its major aspects

so what?

必须 懂得 运用
bìxū dǒngdé yùnyòng

(we) must understand how to employ (something)

what?

八 纲
bā gāng

the eight principles

250

<u>Second unit of meaning</u>

Basic statement

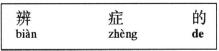

the eight principles are yin and yang, ...

1. Adjunct statement

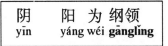

they are **guiding principles**

what guiding
principles?

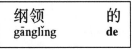

(those) **of** differentiating the pathoconditions

2. Adjunct statement

阴　　阳　为 纲领
yīn　　yáng wéi **gānglǐng**

yin and yang are **guiding principles**

what guiding
principles?

纲领　　　　的
gānglǐng　　　**de**

(those) **of** the guiding principles

where?

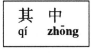

among them

<u>Third unit of meaning</u>

Basic statement

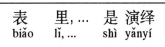

outside/inside, ... are deductions

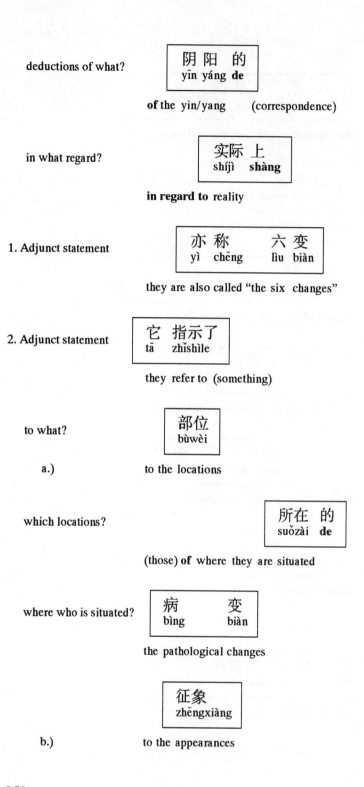

deductions of what?

阴 阳 的
yīn yáng **de**

of the yin/yang　　(correspondence)

in what regard?

实际 上
shíjì **shàng**

in regard to reality

1. Adjunct statement

亦 称　　六 变
yì chēng　liù biàn

they are also called "the six changes"

2. Adjunct statement

它 指示了
tā zhǐshìle

they refer to (something)

to what?

部位
bùwèi

a.)　　　　　　to the locations

which locations?

所在 的
suǒzài **de**

(those) **of** where they are situated

where who is situated?

病　　变
bìng　　biàn

the pathological changes

征象
zhēngxiàng

b.)　　　　　　to the appearances

252

which appearances?

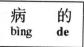

(those) **of** the illnesses

和　変化
hé　biànhuà

c.)　and to changes

what
changes?

消　　長　的
xiāo　zhǎng　de

(those) **of** the waning and waxing

which waning and
waxing?

邪　　正
xíe　zhèng

(those) of evil and proper (qi)

Fourth unit of meaning

Statement

根据　　　八　纲
gēnjù　　　bā　gāng

(we) **base**　(ourself) on the eight principles

why?

来 观察　全部 情况
laí guānchá　quánbù qíngkuàng

to　examine the entire　circumstances

which circumstances?

症　候　的
zhèng　hóu　de

(those) **of** pathological signs

253

and furthermore?

加以 分析　归纳
jiāyǐ fēnxī　guīnà

and add　analysis and deduction

what will happen?

得出 诊断 结论
déchū zhěnduàn jiélùn

(we) reach　diagnostic conclusions

how?

不 难
bù nán

it is not difficult

Fifth unit of meaning

Basic statement

已　叙述
yǐ　xùshù

(we) have already recounted (something)

in what
regard?

关于　阴　阳 方面
guānyù　yīn　yáng **fāngmiàn**

in regard to yin and yang

where?

在　第一 章
zài　dìyī zhāng

in the first　chapter

Adjunct statement

兹　说明　如 下
cī　shuōmíng　rú xià

here (we) explain　something as　follows

what?

意义
yìyì

the meaning

what meaning?

六 变 的
lìu biàn de

(that) of the six changes

255

Text 8.2

Sentence structures

<u>First unit of meaning</u>

Basic statement

表	是	外
biǎo	shì	wài

"outside" is   outer

Adjunct statement

里	是	内
lǐ	shì	nèi

"inside" is   inner

<u>Second unit of meaning</u>

Basic statement

表	是	体	表
biǎo	shì	tǐ	biǎo

the "outside" is   the body's outside

in what
regard?

从	内	外	来	说
cóng	nèi	wài	**lái**	**shūo**

in regard to inner and outer

whose inner
and outer?

人	体	的
rén	tǐ	**de**

(those) **of** the human body

1. Adjunct statement

包括	组织
bāokuò	zǔzhī

(that) includes tissues

which tissues?

皮肤　　肌肉　等
pífū　　jīròu　děng

skin　and muscles

2. Adjunct statement

里　　指　　　内　脏
lǐ　　zhǐ　　　nèi　zàng

the "inside" refers to the inner depots

3. Adjunct statement

包括　　　器官
bāokuò　　qìguān

(that) includes the organs

which organs?

脏,　　腑　　和　　脑　等
zàng,　　fǔ　　hé　　nǎo　děng

the depots, the palaces, and the brain

Third unit of meaning

Basic statement

症　　　　为　表　症
zhèng　　　wéi biǎo zhèng

pathoconditions are outside pathoconditions

which
pathoconditions?

属...者　均
shǔ...zhě　**jūn**

all (those) belonging　　(to something)

what do they
belong to?

于　　体　表
yú　　tǐ　　biǎo

to　the body's outside

for example?

如 恶　　寒, ... 等
rú wù　　hán, ... děng

e.g., aversion to cold, ..

in what regard?

症状
zhèngzhuàng

(in regard of) the pathomanifestations

which patho-
manifestations?

所　出现的
suǒ　chūxiànde

those appearing

when do they appear?

病　邪 侵犯　　人体
bìng xié qīnfàn　　réntǐ

when an illness evil invades the human body

Adjunct statement

症　　为里 症
zhèng　　wéi lǐ zhèng

the pathoconditions are inside pathoconditions

which
pathoconditions?

属　于　体　内　者
shǔ　yú　tǐ　nèi　zhě

those **belonging** to the body's interior

for example?

神　昏　　烦躁, ... 等
shén hūn　　fánzào, ... děng

(e.g.,) mental confusion and restlessness, ...

Text 8.3

Sentence structures

First unit of meaning

Basic statement

邪 侵犯　人　体
xié qīnfàn rén tǐ

the evil invade the human body

which evil?

六淫　　之
liù yín **zhī**

(those) **of** the six excesses

which six excesses?

风, 寒 等
fēng, hán děng

wind, cold, etc.

what will happen?

首先　　伤 于 皮　毛, ...
shǒuxiān shāng yú pí máo, ...

first　(there is) harm to skin and hair, ...

Adjunct statement

概　　称 表 症
gài chēng biǎo zhèng

summarily they are called outside pathoconditions

Second unit of meaning

Basic statement

病　　多 自 内 生
bìng duō zì nèi **shēng**

illnesses **emerge** mostly from the interior

259

which illnesses?

所　　　　引起的
suǒ　　　　yǐnqǐde

those which are brought forth

brought forth
by what?

因　七　情　或　饮　　食…
yīn　qī　qíng　huò yǐn　shí…

by　the seven affects or　drink and food, …

which seven
affects?

喜 怒
xǐ nù

joy, anger etc.

Adjunct statement

概　　　　称　里　症
gài　　　　chēng lǐ　zhèng

summarily they are called inside pathoconditions

Third unit of meaning

Statement

这 是　概况
zhè shì　gàikuàng

that is　a survey

a survey of what?

辨别　　　的
biànbié　　　de

(a survey) **of** a differentiation

a differentiation
of what?

表　里
biǎo　lǐ

(of) outside and inside

260

Fourth unit of meaning

Basic statement

表　邪　可以　传
biǎo　xié　kěyǐ　chuán

an outside evil can　be transmitted

where?

内
nèi

to the interior

Adjunct statement

进　入　脏　腑
jìn　rù　zàng　fǔ

it enters into the depots and palaces

what will happen?

则　症状
zé　zhèngzhuàng

then the pathomanifestations

为 里　症
wéi lǐ　zhèng

are inside pathoconditions

which patho-manifestations?

其 所　现的
qí suǒ　xiànde

those which are manifested by it

Fifth unit of meaning

Basic statement

也 有
yě yǒu

it also happens

what?

表　邪　虽　已　　　传
biǎo　xié　**suí** yǐ　　　chuán

although an outside evil has　　already been transmitted

where?

内
nèi

to the interior

but?

而　　　尚　未　到　　　里
ér　　　shàng **wèi** dào　　　lǐ

but it has **not** yet　　reached the inside

Adjunct statement

成为　半　表　　半　里　症
chéngwéi bàn biǎo　bàn lǐ　zhèng

that is called　　half-outside- half-inside-pathocondition

Sixth unit of meaning

Basic statement

表　邪　内　传
biǎo　xié　**nèi**　chuán

when an outside evil　　is transmitted to the **interior**

and?

表　症　　　仍　在
biǎo　zhèng　　　réng zài

while the outside pathoconditions are still present

what is then?

称为　表　　里　　同　病
chēngwéi biǎo　　lǐ　　tóng　bìng

that is called　　outside and inside are jointly ill

262

<u>Seventh unit of meaning</u>

Basic statement

分辨	表	里	症
fēnbiàn	biǎo	lǐ	zhèng

(we) distinguish outside and inside pathoconditions

in what regard?

临症	上
línzhèng	**shàng**

in regard to clinical   practice

Adjunct statement

更	重要的	是
gèng	zhòngyàode	shì

the **even more** important   (aspect) is

what?

注意	倾向
zhùyì	qīngxiàng

to **pay attention** to the directions

what directions?

其	传	变
qí	chuán	biàn

(those) of their transmission and change

Text 8.4

Sentence structures

<u>First unit of meaning</u>

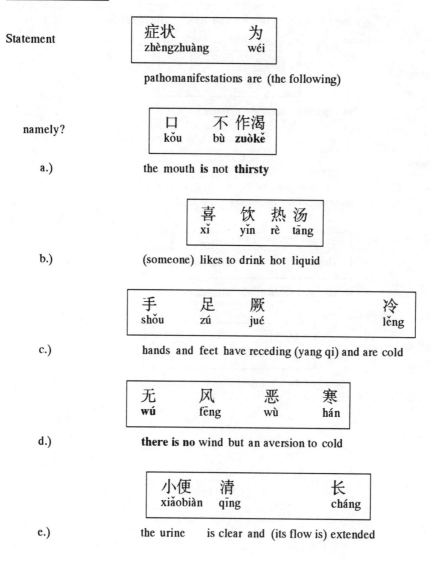

Statement

症状   为
zhèngzhuàng   wéi

pathomanifestations are (the following)

namely?

口   不   作渴
kǒu   bù   **zuòkě**

a.)   the mouth **is not thirsty**

喜   饮   热   汤
xǐ   yǐn   rè   tāng

b.)   (someone) likes to drink hot liquid

手   足   厥   冷
shǒu   zú   jué   lěng

c.)   hands and feet have receding (yang qi) and are cold

无   风   恶   寒
wú   fēng   wù   hán

d.)   **there is no** wind but an aversion to cold

小便   清   长
xiǎobiàn   qīng   cháng

e.)   the urine   is clear and (its flow is) extended

f. - i.: structure identical with e.

264

these are patho-
manifestations
of what?

寒 的
hán **de**

of cold

Second unit of meaning: Structure identical with First unit of meaning

Third unit of meaning

Basic statement

表现　　有　现象
biǎoxiàn　yǒu　xiànxiàng

manifestations have appearances

which manifestations?

病　情　的
bìng　qíng　**de**

a.)　　(those) **of** the illness nature

这里 可以　看出
zhèlǐ kěyǐ　kànchū

b.)　　(those) which　　can　be observed **here**

which
appearances?

两种　　不 同的
liǎngzhǒng bù　tóngde

two　　dis- similar (ones)

appearances
of what?

寒 和 热
hán hé rè

of cold and heat

Adjunct statement

辨别　　是 一个 关键
biànbié　shì yīgè guānjiàn

differentiation is　a　　key element

265

differentiation between
what?

寒　热
hán　rè

between cold and heat

key element of what?

决定　用 药 的
juédìng　yòng yào de

of deciding about using drugs

which drugs?

或　温　或 凉
huò　wēn　huò liáng

whether to use warming or　cooling (drugs)

Fourth unit of meaning

Basic statement

寒 症　和 热 症
hán zhèng　hé rè zhèng

cold pathoconditions and heat pathoconditions

是 全 身 症状
shì quán shēn zhèngzhuàng

are entire body pathomanifestations

always?

有时　不 完全
yǒushí　bù wánquán

sometimes not completely

1. Adjunct statement

如 发热 是　全 身 的
rú fārè shì　quán shēn de

e.g., fever is　(a condition) **of** the entire body

2. Adjunct statement

小溲 可以 有 关
xiǎosōu kěyǐ yǒu guān

urine   can   have relationships

which urine?

黄 赤
huáng chì

yellow red (urine)

relationships
to what?

与 发热
yǔ fārè

to fever

3. Adjunct statement

也 有
yě yǒu

it also happens

what happens?

仅 属 于
jǐn shǔ yú

(fever) does solely belong to (the following condition)

to which condition?

膀胱 有 热
pángguāng yǒu rè

the bladder   has heat

Fifth unit of meaning

Statement

所以 辨 寒 症
suǒyǐ biàn hán zhèng

hence to distinguish cold pathoconditions

267

和 热 症
hé rè zhèng

and heat pathoconditions

what is
to be done?

需要 进一步　　　分别
xūyào jìnyībù　　　fēnbié

(we) must　go a step further and distinguish (something)

what?

上　　下
shàng　xià

upper and lower (locations)

in what regard?

除　　　一般者　　以外
chú　　　yībānzhě　　yǐwài

in addition to the general　(criteria)

Text 8.5

Sentence structures

First unit of meaning

Statement

虚	实	是	说的
xū	shí	shì	shuōde

depletion and repletion are mentioned

what for?

指 ...	来
zhǐ ...	**lái**

to refer to something

what?

两	方面
liǎng	fāngmiàn

two aspects

namely?

正	气	和	邪	气
zhèng	qì	hé	xié	qì

proper qi and evil qi

Second unit of meaning

Basic statement

指	强	弱
zhǐ	qiáng	ruò

they refer to strength and weakness

strength and weakness
of what?

正	气	的
zhèng	qì	**de**

of the proper qi

<table>
<tr><td>in what
regard?</td><td>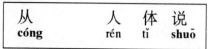</td></tr>
</table>

从	人	体	说
cóng	rén	tǐ	shuō

in regard to the human body

Adjunct statement: Structure identical with basic statement

Third unit of meaning

Basic statement

虚	多	指	正	气
xū	duō	zhǐ	zhèng	qì

depletion often refers to proper qi

where?

在	一般	临症	上
zài	yībān	línzhèng	shàng

in general clinical practice

1. Adjunct statement: Structure identical with basic statement

2. Adjunct statement

因
yīn

the reason (is the following)

namely?

正	气	充旺
zhèng	qì	chōngwàng

proper qi flourishes

and?

无	所	谓	实
wú	suǒ	wèi	shí

nothing exists that is to be called repletion

270

3. Adjunct statement

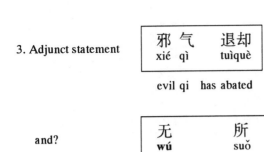

evil qi has abated

and?

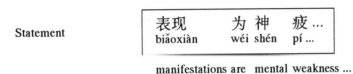

nothing exists that is to be called depletion

Fourth unit of meaning

Statement

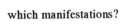

manifestations are mental weakness ...

which manifestations?

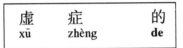

(those) **of** the depletion pathoconditions

Fifth unit of meaning: Structure identical with Fourth unit of meaning

Sixth unit of meaning

Basic statement

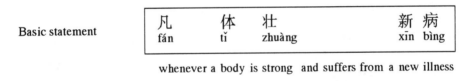

whenever a body is strong and suffers from a new illness

what is then?

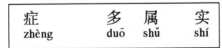

the pathoconditions mostly belong to repletion

Adjunct statement: structure identical with Basic statement

Basic statement

体	质		和	机转	表现	为
tǐ	zhì		hé	jīzhuǎn	biǎoxiàn	wéi

physical constitution and processes appear   as   (something)

whose constitution?

患者
huànzhě

(that) of the patient

which processes?

病理
bìnglǐ

the pathological (ones)

they appear
as what?

有	余		结实,...	的
yǒu	yú		jiéshí, ...	de

as having surplus, being firm, ...   ones

what is then?

称为	实	症
chēngwèi shí		zhèng

they are called   repletion pathoconditions

Adjunct statement: structure identical with Basic statement

Text 8.6

Sentence structures

<u>First unit of meaning</u>

Statement

辨别	是	根据
biànbié	shì	gēnjù

to differentiate is   the basis

to differentiate
what?

虚	实
xū	shí

depletion and repletion

is the basis
of what?

攻	邪 和	补	正	的
gōng	xié hé	bǔ	zhèng	de

of attacking evil and of supplementing proper (qi)

<u>Second unit of meaning</u>

Basic statement

病	有	纯	虚...	者
bìng	**yǒu**	chún	xū...	**zhě**

if there is, as illness,   pure depletion...

what is then?

辨别	较	易
biànbié	jiào	yì

to differentiate is relatively easy

and?

治疗	亦	简单
zhìliáo	yì	jiǎndān

to treat   is also easy

1. Adjunct statement

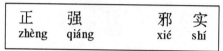

有	虚	实	错杂 者
yǒu	xū	shí	cuòzá zhě

if there is depletion and repletion mixed

能	挽救
néng	wǎnjìu

it is possible to help

when?

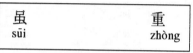

正	强	邪	实
zhèng	qiáng	xié	shí

if the proper is strong, and if the evil is weak

under all
circumstances?

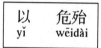

虽	重
sūi	zhòng

although (the condition) is serious

2. Adjunct statement

以	危殆
yǐ	wēidài

it can also be dangerous

when?

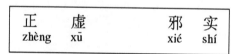

正	虚	邪	实
zhèng	xū	xié	shí

if the proper is depleted while the evil is replete

under all
circumstances?

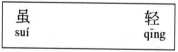

虽	轻
suí	qīng

although (the problem) is light

274

Third unit of meaning

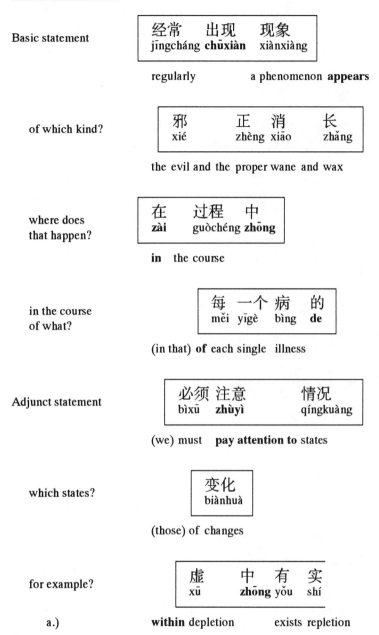

Basic statement	经常　　出现　　现象 jīngcháng **chūxiàn** xiànxiàng regularly　　a phenomenon **appears**	
of which kind?	邪　　正　消　　长 xié　　zhèng xiāo　　zhǎng the evil and the proper wane and wax	
where does that happen?	在　　过程　　中 **zài**　guòchéng **zhōng** **in**　the course	
in the course of what?	每　一个　病　　的 měi　yīgè　bìng　**de** (in that) **of** each single illness	
Adjunct statement	必须 注意　　　情况 bìxū　**zhùyì**　qíngkuàng (we) must　**pay attention to** states	
which states?	变化 biànhuà (those) of changes	
for example?	虚　中　有　实 xū　**zhōng** yǒu shí	
a.)	**within** depletion　　exists repletion	

275

实	中	有	虚
shí	**zhōng**	yǒu	xū

within repletion   exists depletion

虚	多	实	少, ...
xū	duō	shí	shǎo, ...

b.)   depletion is more, repletion is less, ...

Fourth unit of meaning

Basic statement

例如
lìrú

for example (the following conditions)

namely?

外	感	风	寒
wài	gǎn	fēng	hán

a.)   external affection by wind cold

恶	寒	发热
wù	hán	fārè

b.)   aversion to cold with fever

脉	象	浮	紧
mài	xiàng	fú	jǐn

c.)   the pulse appears superficial and tight

what is that?

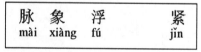

这	是	一个	表	实	症
zhè	shì	yīgè	biǎo	shí	zhèng

that is an   outside-repletion pathocondition

1. Adjunct statement

如果 汗 出 不 止
rúguǒ hàn chū bù zhǐ

if   sweat flows without end

when?

发 汗 后
fā hàn hòu

after (we) have induced sweating

and?

身 热 骤 降
shēn rè zòu jiàng

a.)   the body heat suddenly drops

反 而 畏
fǎn ér wèi

b.)   **and**, in contrast,   (we) fear (something)

what?

冷 更 剧
lěng gèng jù

the cooling down even worsens

what is that?

这 是 症 象
zhè shì zhèng xiàng

that is   a pathological sign

sign of what?

转 为 虚 症
zhuǎn wèi xū zhèng

of a change into a depletion pathocondition

2. Adjunct statement: structure identical with 1. Adjunct statement

277

Text 8.7

Sentence structures

<u>First unit of meaning</u>

Basic statement

表	里, ...	是	一	种	归纳	方法
biǎo	lǐ, ...	shì	yī	zhǒng	guīnà	fāngfǎ

outside/inside, ... are a kind of classifying method

for the classi-
fication of what?

症状	的
zhèngzhuàng	**de**

of the pathomanifestations

Adjunct statement

单	看	一个	症状
dān	kàn	yīge	zhèngzhuàng

to only observe one pathomanifestation

是	没有意思的
shì	méiyǒuyìsīde

is meaningless

<u>Second unit of meaning</u>

Basic statement

因为	每一个	症状	都	能	出现
yīnwèi	**měiyīge**	zhèngzhuàng	**dōu**	néng	chūxiàn

the reason is, **each** pathomanifestation can appear

how can it appear?

在	两	方面
zài	liǎng	fāngmiàn

in two aspects

1. Adjunct statement

表	症	有	怕	冷
biǎo	zhèng	yǒu	pà	lěng

outside pathoconditions include aversion to cold

2. - 6. Adjunct statement: structure identical with 1. Adjunct statement

Third unit of meaning

Statement

究竟	属	于	哪一	类型?
jiūjìng	shǔ	yú	nǎyī	lèixíng?

finally it belongs to which type?

Fourth unit of meaning

Statement

必须	结合	多种	症状
bìxū	jiéhé	duōzhǒng	zhèngzhuàng

(we) must combine many pathomanifestations

why?

来	决定
lái	juédìng

to decide (this)

Fifth unit of meaning

Basic statement

所以	分析
suǒyǐ	fēnxī

hence (we) analyze (something)

what?

把	许多	症状	加以
bǎ	xǔduō	zhèngzhuàng	jiāyǐ

many pathomanifestations

279

1. Adjunct statement

就　　联系起来
jìu　　liánxìqǐlái

then (we) combine

what?

类同
lèitóng

similar (ones)

similar in what regard?

其　性质　上的
qí　xìngzhì　**shàngde**

in regard to their nature

2. Adjunct statement

成为　一个　群
chéngwéi yīge　qún

(we) form　one　group

a group of what?

症候
zhènghòu

of patho-indicators

3. Adjunct statement

才　　能　诊断
cái　　néng zhěnduàn

then (we) can　diagnose

what?

它是　表　　是　里, ...
tā　shì　biǎo　shì　lǐ, ...

it　is　an outside or it is　an inside (problem)

280

<u>Sixth unit of meaning</u>

Basic statement

这 说明了
zhè shuōmíngle

this explains   (something)

what?

目的是 在 求   本 质
mùdì shì zài qíu   běn zhì

the goal   is   in   searching for the basic nature

goal of what?

辨   症   的
biàn   zhèng   **de**

of differentiating pathoconditions

what basic nature?

病   的
bìng   **de**

(that) **of** an illness

Adjunct statement

要   掌握   真相
yào   zhǎngwò   zhēnxiàng

(we) wish to grasp   the truth

what is then?

必须 观察
bìxū guānchá

(we) must   examine (a problem)

how?

从 多 方面
cóng duō fāngmiàn

from many sides

Text 8.8

Sentence structures

First unit of meaning

Basic statement

内容	包括了	关系
nèiróng	bāokuòle	guānxì

the contents comprise the relationships

what contents?

八	纲	的
bā	gāng	**de**

(those) **of** the eight principles

principles of what?

辨	症
biàn	zhèng

(those) of differentiating the pathoconditions

which relationships?

体	表	和	体	内	的
tǐ	biǎo	hé	tǐ	nèi	**de**

(those) **of** the body's outside and of the body's inside

1. Adjunct statement

指出了	性质 和	情况
zhǐchūle	xìngzhì hé	qíngkuàng

they refer to the nature and to the circumstances

circumstances of what?

发展
fāzhǎn

(those) of the development

what nature and developmental circumstances?

病	症	的
bìng	zhèng	**de**

(those) **of** illness-conditions

282

Second unit of meaning

Basic statement

<table>
<tr><td>最后</td><td>阶段</td><td>是</td><td>为了</td><td>治疗</td></tr>
<tr><td>zuìhòu</td><td>jiēduàn</td><td>shì</td><td>wèile</td><td>zhìliáo</td></tr>
</table>

the final phase is **devoted to** therapy

what final phase?

<table>
<tr><td>辨</td><td>症</td><td>的</td></tr>
<tr><td>biàn</td><td>zhèng</td><td>de</td></tr>
</table>

(that) **of** differentiating pathoconditions

1. Adjunct statement

<table>
<tr><td>分辨</td><td>表</td><td>里</td></tr>
<tr><td>fēnbiàn</td><td>biǎo</td><td>lǐ</td></tr>
</table>

(we) distinguish outside and inside

what for?

<table>
<tr><td>可以</td><td>定出</td></tr>
<tr><td>kěyǐ</td><td>dìngchū</td></tr>
</table>

(we) can decide (something)

what?

<table>
<tr><td>或</td><td>汗</td><td>或</td><td>下</td></tr>
<tr><td>huò</td><td>hàn</td><td>huò</td><td>xià</td></tr>
</table>

whether to cause sweating or to purge

2. and 3. Adjunct statement: structure identical with 1. Adjunct statement

Third unit of meaning

Basic statement

<table>
<tr><td>汗</td><td>法</td><td>有</td><td>辛</td><td>温</td><td>发汗, ...</td></tr>
<tr><td>hàn</td><td>fǎ</td><td>yǒu</td><td>xīn</td><td>wēn</td><td>fāhàn, ...</td></tr>
</table>

the sweating pattern includes acrid and warming diaphoresis, ...

1. Adjunct statement: structure identical with Basic statement

283

2. Adjunct statement

其它	也	都	有	不	同的	用	法
qítā	yě	dōu	yǒu	bù	tóngde	yòng	fǎ

the other, too, all have dis- similar application patterns

which others?

温	法,	凉	法, ...
wēn	fǎ,	liáng	fǎ, ...

the warming pattern, the cooling pattern, ...

Fourth unit of meaning

Basic statement

如何来	确定	治疗	方针
rúhélái	quèdìng	zhìliáo	fāngzhēn

how   to determine a therapeutic approach?

which therapeutic approach?

具体的
jùtǐde

a specific (one)

Adjunct statement

非	结合	不	可
fēi	jiéhé	bù	kě

without combining, it is not possible

without combining what?

表	里,	寒	热,	虚	实
biǎo	lǐ,	hán	rè,	xū	shí

outside and inside, cold and heat, depletion and repletion

Stroke Order of Characters

Text 1.1

中	丨	冂	口	中			
医	一	丆	歹	医	医	医	医
用	丿	门	月	月	用		
阴	阝	阝	阴	阴	阴	阴	
阳	阝	阝	阳	阳	阳	阳	
学	丷	丷	兯	兯	学	学	学
说	丶	讠	讠	讠	讠	诮	诮
	说	说					
来	一	一	平	平	未	来	来
明	丨	冂	日	日	旧	明	明
	明						
上	丨	上	上				
的	丿	白	白	白	白	的	的

285

Text 1.1

的						
一	十	卄	甘	甚	其	其
其	基	基	基			
一	十	才	木	本		
丶	亻	门	问	问	问	
丨	冂	日	旦	早	是	昰
是	是	是	是	题	题	题
题						
丿	人	从	从			
一	丆	厅	雨	而	而	
一	厂	厉	成	成	成	
丶	丿	为	为			
一	三	玉	珡	珇	珇	理

286

Stroke Order of Characters

Text 1.1

	理	理	理	理		
论思	⺀	讠	讠	论	论	
	⺀	冂	曰	田	思	思
	思	思				
想	二	十	才	木	机	机	相
	相	相	相	想	想	想
体系它贯	⺀	亻	仁	什	休	休	体
	乙	纟	乡	玉	系	系	系
	丶	宀	宀	宀	它		
	⺀	冂	毌	毌	毌	贯	贯
	贯	贯					
串在	⺀	冂	吕	吕	吕	吕	串
	一	十	才	在	在	在

Text 1.1

生	ノ	一	生	生	生		
病	丶	亠	广	疒	疒	疗	疔
	病	病	病				
诊	丶	讠	讠	诊	诊	诊	诊
断	丶	丷	半	米	米	断	
	断	断	断	断			
治	丶	氵	氵	泸	沿	治	治
	治						
疗	丶	亠	广	广	疒	疗	
和	二	二	禾	禾	禾	和	和
	和						
药	一	卅	卅	药	药	药	药
	药	药					

Stroke Order of Characters

Text 1.1

物	⺧	㇆	牛	牛	牪	物	物
	物						
等	⺧	㇆	㇕	竹	竹	竺	笁
	筜	笁	等	等	等		
各	⺧	夕	冬	各	各	各	
个	⺧	人	个				
方	⺀	亠	立	方			
面	一	丆	西	丙	面	而	面
	面	面					
构	一	十	才	木	杓	杓	构
	构						
了	了						
整	一	二	丙	車	束	束	束

Text 1.1

	敕	敕	敕	敕	整	整	整
	整	整					
套	一	大	大	杏	杏	套	套
	套	套	套				
合	ノ	人	今	合	合	合	
乎	ノ	⺊	⺈	乒	乎		
客	⺍	⺍	宀	宏	岁	客	客
	客	客					
观	刀	双	观	观	观	观	
实	⺍	⺍	宀	宓	宝	实	实
	实						
际	阝	阝	阝	际	阽	际	际
法	⺀	⺀	氵	氵	沽	法	法

290

Text 1.1

	法						
灵	⁊	⁊	彐	彐	灵	灵	灵
活	丶	冫	氵	沪	泸	活	活
	活	活					
地	一	十	土	圹	地	地	
指	一	十	扌	护	护	指	指
	指	指					
导	⁊	⁊	彐	与	导	导	
着	丷	丷	丷	兰	兰	兰	养
	养	着	着	着			
临	⎪	リ	リ	リ	リ	临	临
	临	临					
床	丶	亠	广	庐	庁	牙	床

Text 1.1

践	ㄣ	ㄦ	卫	무	몸	尻	足
	趵	趵	践	践	践		

Stroke Order of Characters

Text 1.2

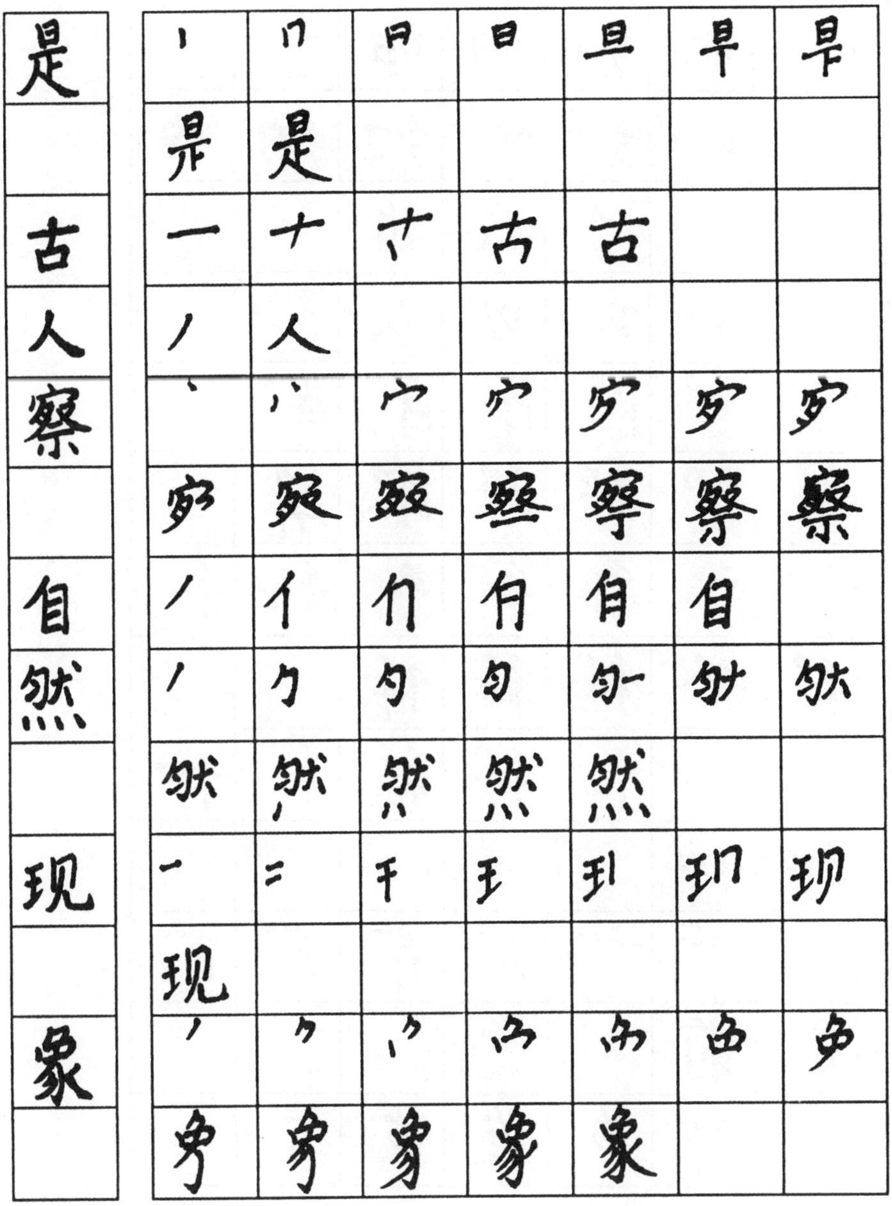

是	丶	冂	冃	日	旦	早	畢
	是	是					
古	一	十	士	古	古		
人	丿	人					
察	丶	八	宀	宀	穸	穸	穸
	穸	寂	寂	蔡	寧	察	察
自	丿	亻	什	自	自	自	
然	丿	夕	夕	匀	勾一	�	然
	然	然	然	然	然		
现	一	二	干	王	玡	玥	现
	现						
象	丿	ク	冷	凸	凸	由	多
	多	象	象	象	象		

293

Text 1.2

归	⼁	⼅	⼮⼅	⼮⼅	归		
纳	⼂	⼦	⼦	纟	幻	纳	纳
出	⼄	山	屵	屵	出		
以	⼁	⼂	⼂	以	以		
解	⼃	⼇	广	冇	角	角	角
	角	角	解	解	解	解	
释	⼃	⼂	⼫	丷	平	禾	釆
	釆	釈	釈	释	释		
种	⼃	⼆	千	千	禾	和	和
	和	种					
前	⼂	丷	丷	广	首	首	首
	前	前					
发	⼄	⼩	发	发	发		

294

Text 1.2

万	一	丁	万				
都	一	十	土	耂	老	者	者
	者	都	都				
有	一	ナ	𠂇	有	有	有	
正	一	丁	下	正	正		
反	丿	厂	反	反			
两	一	冂	两	两	两	两	两
属	一	𡰣	尸	尸	屈	居	居
	居	属	属	属			
性	丶	忄	忄	忄	忄	性	性
	性						
这	丶	二	亍	文	文	讠	这
对	丿	又	𰀪	对	对		

Text 1.2

立	丶	亠	六	立	立		
又	フ	又					
统	乚	纟	纟	纟	红	红	统
	纺	统					
普	丶	业	半	並	並	並	並
	並	普	普	普	普		
遍	丶	宀	户	户	尸	启	启
	扁	扁	编	遍	遍		
存	一	ナ	才	存	存		
于	一	二	于				
切	一	七	切	切			
事	一	匚	甴	写	弓	写	昌
	事						

Text 1.2

就	丶	亠	六	亩	亡	亨	京
	京	京	計	就	就		
创	丿	人	今	仓	创	创	
名	丿	夕	夕	夕	名	名	
词	丶	讠	讦	词	词	词	词
代	丿	亻	仁	代	代		
表	一	二	丰	丰	声	丰	表
	表						
所	丶	厂	斤	戶	所	所	所
	所						
关	丶	丷	兰	兰	关	关	
如	乀	女	女	如	如	如	
天	一	二	于	天			

Text 1.2

日	丨	冂	日	日			
月	丿	刀	月	月			
昼	乛	コ	尸	尺	尺	尽	昼
	昼	昼					
夜	丶	亠	广	疒	疒	疗	夜
	夜						
火	丶	丷	少	火			
水	丨	刀	水	水			
并	丶	丷	丷	兰	羊	并	
相	一	十	才	木	朾	相	相
	相	相					
道	丶	丷	䒑	䒑	䒑	首	首
	首	首	首	道	道		

Stroke Order of Characters

Text 1.2

去	一	十	土	去	去		
宇	丶	宀	宀	亠	宇		
宙	丶	宀	宀	宀	宁	宁	宙
	宙						
间	丶	门	门	门	问	间	间
变	丶	亠	宁	亦	亦	亦	变
	变						
化	丿	亻	化	化			

Text 1.3

认	丶	讠	讥	认			
也	乛	力	也				
能	ㄥ	厶	乍	自	自	自	能
	能	能	能				
加	乛	力	加	加	加		
般	丿	亻	介	舟	舟	舟	舟
	舠	船	般				
质	丿	厂	斤	斥	斥	质	质
	质						
动	一	二	云	云	云丁	动	
静	一	二	丰	丰	丰	青	青
	青	青	青	静	静	静	静
保	丿	亻	伫	伫	伻	伻	

Stroke Order of Characters

Text 1.3

	保	保					
卫	フ	ア	卫				
力	フ	力					
守	丶	宀	宀	宁	守	守	
内	丨	冂	内	内			
部	丶	亠	立	立	立	产	音
	音	部	部				
精	丶	丷	丷	半	米	米	米
	米	料	精	精	精	精	精
气	丿	仁	乞	气			
作	丿	亻	化	化	作	作	作
故	一	十	古	古	古	古	故
	故	故					

Text 1.3

皮	⁻	厂	广	皮	皮		
毛	⸌	⸗	三	毛			
肌	丿	刀	月	月	肌	肌	
肉	⸌	冂	内	内	肉	肉	
筋	丿	⸌	⸗	⸗	⸗	⸗	广
	竺	筝	筝	筋	筋		
骨	⸜	冖	冂	冎	骨	骨	骨
	骨	骨					
脏	丿	刀	月	月	月	肜	肜
	脏	脏	脏				
腑	丿	刀	月	月	月	肜	肜
	肜	肜	肜	腑	腑		
五	一	丁	五	五			

302

Stroke Order of Characters

Text 1.3

主藏	丶	亠	二	宁	主		
	一	十	艹	芏	芦	疒	疒
	疒	疒	芲	菀	菧	藏	藏
	藏	藏	藏				
司消	刁	刁	司	司	司		
	丶	冫	氵	氵	沙	沙	沙
	消	消	消				
传位	丿	亻	仁	仁	传	传	
位置	丿	亻	亻	位	位	位	位
	丶	冂	四	四	四	罒	罒
	罒	罘	罟	胃	置	置	
分焦	丿	八	分	分			
	丿	亻	亻	仁	仁	信	隹

Text 1.3

	佳	佳	隹	焦	焦		
外	丿	夕	夕	列	外		
侧	丿	亻	侧	们	侧	侧	侧
	侧						
功	一	丁	工	功	功		
血	丿	亻	仃	血	血	血	
每	丿	仁	乞	每	每	每	每
处	丿	夕	夂	处	处		
特	丿	仁	牛	牛	牛	牛	牛
	牛	特	特				
殊	一	丆	歹	歹	列	歼	死
	殊	殊	殊				

Text 1.4

根	一	十	才	木	杠	村	柯
	根	根	根				
据	一	十	才	扩	护	护	护
	捉	捉	据	据			
区	一	匚	匚	区			
别	丶	口	口	号	另	别	别
症	丶	亠	广	广	疒	疒	疔
	疔	疔	症				
里	丶	冂	日	日	旦	甲	里
热	一	十	才	扌	执	执	热
	热	热	热				
寒	丶	八	宀	宀	宀	宫	宝
	宝	寎	寒	寒			

305

Text 1.4

凡	ノ	几	凡				
机	一	十	才	木	机	机	
衰	丶	一	亠	亠	亩	音	亭
	衰	衰	衰				
弱	フ	コ	弓	弓	弓	弓	弓
	弱	弱	弱				
少	ノ	小	小	少			
懶	丶	丨	忄	忄	忄	忄	忄
	悚	悚	悚	懶	懶	懶	懶
	懶	懶					
言	丶	亠	亠	言	言	言	言
怕	丶	丨	忄	忄	忄	怕	怕
	怕						

306

Text 1.4

冷	、	冫	冫	冷	冷	冷	冷
疲	、	亠	广	广	疒	疒	疒
	疒	疖	疲				
倦	丿	亻	伫	伫	伫	伴	伴
	佯	佯	倦				
不	一	丆	才	不			
耐	一	丆	而	丙	而	而	而
	耐	耐					
劳	一	十	艹	艹	芍	劳	劳
多	丿	夕	夕	多	多	多	
足	、	口	口	早	足	足	足
损	一	才	扌	护	护	护	
	损	损	损				

Text 1.4

失	ノ	⸠	上	生	失		
贫	ノ	八	分	分	分	贫	贫
	贫						
姜	一	丷	艹	艹	兰	芏	羊
	来	姜	姜	姜			
黄	一	艹	艹	芏	艹	苦	昔
	苗	苗	黄	黄			
遗	丶	冂	口	中	虫	虫	串
	贵	贵	贵	遗	遗		
瘦	丶	亠	广	广	疒	疒	疒
	疒	疬	疬	疬	瘦	瘦	
因	丨	门	冂	囚	因	因	
把	一	十	才	扣	扣	扣	把

Text 1.4

状	、	ン	⺥	⺦	⺦	状	状
四	、	冂	四	四	四		
类	丶	⺮	丷	半	半	米	米
	关	类					
型	一	二	干	开	刑	刑	型
	型	型					
即	𠃌	ヨ	ヨ	艮	艮	即	即
虚	丨	上	上	广	卢	虍	虎
	虎	虚	虚	虚			
盛	一	厂	厈	成	成	成	成
	盛	盛	盛	盛			
概	一	十	才	木	杓	杓	杓
	根	根	根	概	概	概	

Text 1.4

括	一	十	扌	扩	扩	括	括
	括	括					
亢	丶	二	广	亢			
进	一	二	扌	井	讲	讲	进
兴	丶	丷	丷	兴	兴	兴	
奋	一	𠂇	大	大	夲	夲	奋
	奋						
倾	丿	亻	化	化	伫	伫	倾
	倾	倾	倾				
向	丿	亻	门	向	向	向	
潜	丶	冫	氵	汇	汇	泸	泱
	汱	泧	潎	潆	潜	潜	潜
	潜						

Text 1.4

伏	丿	亻	亻	什	伏	伏	
推	一	十	扌	扌	扌	扩	扩
	扌	扌	推	推			
至	一	乙	云	互	至	至	
科	丿	二	千	禾	禾	禾	禾
	禾	科					
红	乙	纟	纟	纟	红	红	
肿	丿	刀	月	月	肝	肝	肝
	肿						
白	丿	亻	亻	白	白		
陷	了	阝	阝	阝	阝	阝	阝
	陷	陷	陷				

GENERAL GLOSSARY

A

A 是指 B 来说的	A shì zhǐ B lái shuō de	lit. "A is spoken (i.e., used) to point (i.e., refer) to B;" A refer(s) to B	8.5
A 为 B 所	A wéi B suǒ ...	passive construction: A is ... by B	2.2
哀	āi	grief	5.2
嗳气	ǎi-qì	belching	10.7
安	ān	quiet; peaceful	12.2
安定	ān-dìng	calm	11.8
安神	ān-shén	pacify the spirit	5.6
谙	ān	be familiar with something	11.5
按	àn	press; feel (the pulse)	11.1
按	àn	in accordance with; according to	2.5
按照	àn-zhào	in accordance with	2.8
案	àn	case record	15.6
黯淡	àn-dàn	dim	10.1
熬	áo	boil (slowly with gentle heat)	15.3
熬炼	áo-liàn	boil	15.3

B

八	bā	eight	10.8
八法	bā-fǎ	the eight patterns	13.1
八纲	bā-gāng	the eight principles	8.1
八阵	bā-zhèn	the eight strategic arrays	14.7

把	bǎ	(particle identifying the immediately following expression as an object of the subsequent verb)	1.4
把 A 加以 B	bǎ A jiā yǐ B	(structure indicating that A is an object of B)	8.7
白	bái	white	1.4
白滑	bái-huá	white glossy	8.4
白酒	bái-jiǔ	alcohol	15.4
百	bǎi	hundred	5.2
百数十家	bǎi-shù-shí-jiā	many authors	9.8
般	bān	kind; type	15.8
伴有	bàn-yǒu	be accompanied by	9.2
半表半里	bàn-biǎo-bàn-lǐ	half-outside-half-inside	9.3
半表半里症	bàn-biǎo-bàn-lǐ-zhèng	half-outside-half-inside pathocondition	8.3
半固体	bàn-gù-tǐ	semisolid	15.3
半身不遂	bàn-shēn-bù-suí	hemiplegia	6.2
半夏	bàn-xià	(drug name) Pinellia ternata (Thub.) Breit.	16.2
办法	bàn-fǎ	measure; method	12.5
帮助	bāng-zhù	assist	4.7
胞	bāo	bladder	5.7
包	bāo	wrap	15.5
包含	bāo-hán	include	14.8
包括	bāo-kuò	include	1.8
包括 … 在内	bāo-kuò … zài nèi	include	15.6
保	bǎo	protect	5.7
保持	bǎo-chí	maintain	3.4
保全	bǎo-quán	preserve	16.1
保守	bǎo-shǒu	protect; maintain	1.3
保卫	bǎo-wèi	safeguard; protect	1.3
保证	bǎo-zhèng	guarantee	16.1
饱	bǎo	full (after eating); bloated	7.4

饱满	bǎo-mǎn	(feeling of) fullness	13.2
悲	bēi	sorrow	7.1
悲哀	bēi-āi	grief	7.1
北	běi	north	2.5
背	bèi	back	5.6
背脊	bèi-jǐ	back	3.7
背痛	bèi-tòng	back pain	5.5
贝母	bèi-mǔ	(drug name) Fritillaria cirrhosa D. Don.	16.1
倍	bèi	double; multiply	15.2
被	bèi	(passive pronoun)	4.3
被用	bèi-yòng	be used	9.1
贲门	bēn-mén	lit: "rushing gate"; upper stomach opening	5.7
奔走	bēn-zǒu	walk	6.4
本	běn	origin; originally	2.4
本来	běn-lái	originally	12.8
本身	běn-shēn	itself	2.4
本身	běn-shēn	by nature	7.4
本质	běn-zhì	basic nature	8.7
愊愊然	bī-bī-rán	pressing; forceful	11.2
鼻	bí	nose	2.6
鼻孔	bí-kǒng	nostril	7.5
鼻衄	bí-nǜ	nosebleed	5.7
鼻塞	bí-sè	nasal blockage	3.7
比	bǐ	in comparison to	9.4
比较	bǐ-jiào	relative	9.8
比较	bǐ-jiào	compare with	15.7
比如	bǐ-rú	for example	2.4
毕竟	bì-jìng	finally; in the final analysis	7.2
痹	bì	paralysis	10.5
痹	bì	stiffness	15.4

闭	bì	closure	13.2
闭结	bì-jié	constipation	4.6
必	bì	must; inevitably	2.3
必然	bì-rán	definitely	15.8
必须	bì-xū	must	1.8
必要	bì-yào	necessary; essential	2.3
必由	bì-yóu	essential; necessary	3.3
臂	bì	arm	10.5
避	bì	avoid	10.6
避免	bì-miǎn	avoid	14.1
髀	bì	upper thigh	3.5
便	biàn	(particle indicating that the fact referred to next results from a fact mentioned immediately before)	2.6
便	biàn	easy; facilitate	11.5
便闭	biàn-bì	constipation	6.6
便秘	biàn-bì	constipation	9.2
便溺	biàn-niào	urine	3.5
便是	biàn-shì	(final particle emphasizing the preceding statement)	14.5
便血	biàn-xuè	blood-stools	4.6
变	biàn	change	1.5
变端	biàn-duān	change	10.1
变化	biàn-huà	change	1.2
变为	biàn-wéi	change to	16.2
辨	biàn	differentiate; differentiation	3.4
辨别	biàn-bié	distinguish	8.3
辨认	biàn-rèn	distinguish	16.6
辨症论治	biàn-zhèng-lùn-zhì	determine a therapy on the basis of a differentiation of (a patient's) pathoconditions	3.4

辨症	biàn-zhèng	the differentiation of the pathoconditions	8.1
辨症法	biàn-zhèng-fǎ	pattern to distinguish between pathoconditions	14.4
遍	biàn	everywhere	9.5
标	biāo	tip	12.4
标本	biāo-běn	tip and root	12.4
标症	biāo-zhèng	tip pathocondition	12.7
标志	biāo-zhì	characteristic; reference point	11.1
表	biǎo	exterior; outer side	1.3
表寒	biǎo-hán	outside cold	11.4
表里同病	biǎo-lǐ-tóng-bìng	joint illness outside and inside	8.3
表面上	biǎo-miàn-shàng	on the surface	12.2
表面上	biǎo-miàn-shàng	outside	12.5
表热	biǎo-rè	exterior heat	13.5
表热（症）	biǎo-rè-(zhèng)	(pathocondition of) exterior heat	13.5
表实症	biǎo-shí-zhèng	pathocondition of outside repletion	8.6
表示	biǎo-shì	indicate; be a sign of	11.6
表现	biǎo-xiàn wéi	become manifest as	6.6
表邪	biǎo-xié	outside evil	8.3
表症	biǎo-zhèng	pathoconditions affecting the body's exterior	1.4
别	bié	additional	13.8
别	bié	distinguish	11.5
别出	bié-chū	offshoots	3.2
瘪	biě	shrivelled	10.4
冰片	bīng-piàn	borneol	15.2
丙	bǐng	third (in an enumeration)	2.8
病	bìng	illness	1.4
病变	bìng-biàn	pathological change	1.5
病根	bìng-gēn	root of an illness	12.2

病理	bìng-lǐ	pathology	1.1
病例	bìng-lì	a case of illness	3.4
病名	bìng-míng	illness name	5.3
病气	bìng-qì	qi (odors) emitted by an illness	10.6
病情	bìng-qíng	illness	7.1
病人	bìng-rén	sick person; patient	7.2
病势	bìng-shì	the strength of an illness	10.1
病所	bìng-suǒ	location of an illness	16.8
病体	bìng-tǐ	physical condition during an illness	13.2
病邪	bìng-xié	pathogenic evil	4.2
病因	bìng-yīn	cause of illness	6.1
病症	bìng-zhèng	pathocondition	2.7
病状	bìng-zhuàng	appearance of an illness	6.8
并	bìng	simultaneous	1.2
并	bìng	together	4.1
并	bìng	(particle emphasizing the following negation)	4.8
并病	bìng-bìng	joint illnesses	9.7
并提	bìng-tí	refer together	5.7
并行不悖	bìng-xíng-bù-bèi	move in parallel without contact; coexist without affecting each other	2.3
并用	bìng-yòng	apply simultaneously; simultaneous application	14.6
剥苔	bō-tāi	peeling coating	10.4
薄	bó	thin	10.3
薄弱	bó-ruò	weak	7.4
博	bó	in large measure; comprehensively	14.4
搏	bó	struggle	12.1
补	bǔ	supplement	2.8
补充	bǔ-chōng	supplement	13.8

补法	bǔ-fǎ	method of supplementing	8.8
补剂	bǔ-jì	supplementing remedy	12.2
补气	bǔ-qì	supplement the qi	5.6
补气药	bǔ-qì-yào	drug supplementing qi	5.3
补血	bǔ-xuè	supplement the blood	13.8
补养剂	bǔ-yǎng-jì	supplementing and nourishing prescription	14.8
补养	bǔ-yǎng	tonify	13.8
补药	bǔ-yào	supplementing drug	16.4
补阵	bǔ-zhèn	supplementing array	14.7
不	bù	not	1.4
不安	bù-ān	restless; unquiet	6.7
不但	bù-dàn	not only	13.2
不但 ... 而	bù-dàn ... ér	not only ..., but ...	2.4
不等	bù-děng	not identical	14.6
不定	bù-dìng	unstable	10.1
不断	bù-duàn	continuous	14.4
不过	bù-guò	however	1.8
不及	bù-jí	insufficient	2.4
不禁	bù-jīn	uncontrolled	4.7
不仅	bù-jǐn	not only	3.8
不仅 ... 并 ...	bù-jǐn ... bìng ...	not only ..., but also ...	4.2
不仅 ... 而且 ...	bù-jǐn ... ér-qiě ...	not only ... also ...	14.4
不可	bù-kě	cannot	4.8
不乐	bù-lè	discontent	7.1
不利	bù-lì	impeded flow; blockage of a passage	4.7
不利于	bù-lì-yú	not conducive to	16.2
不良	bù-liáng	not good; bad	6.5
不乱	bù-luàn	not in disorder	10.1
不论	bù-lùn	regardless	1.8

不内外因	bù-nèi-wài-yīn	neither internal nor external causes	6.1
不平	bù-píng	imbalance	16.6
不全面	bù quán-miàn	incomplete	3.8
不胜	bù-shèng	not to win	2.4
不舒	bù-shū	tense	5.6
不同	bù-tóng	different	1.8
不问	bù-wèn	regardless whether	6.8
不省人事	bù-xǐng-rén-shì	recognize neither people nor things	6.2
不醒	bù-xǐng	unconscious	3.5
不一	bù-yī	different	13.4
不一定	bù-yī-dìng	not necessarily	14.2
不宜	bù-yí	should not	12.7
不予	bù-yǔ	not to grant	12.7
不约	bù-yuē	unrestrained	4.7
不再	bù-zài	not again; not any longer	7.2
不止	bù-zhǐ	incessantly	8.6
不足	bù-zú	insufficient	1.4
部	bù	region	10.2
部分	bù-fèn	element	3.1
部位	bù-wèi	location	1.4

C

才	cái	then	1.8
采	cǎi	collect	14.4
采集	cǎi-jí	collect; harvest; gather	16.1
采集时期	cǎi-jí-shí-qī	time of collection	16.1

采取	cǎi-qǔ	select	11.1
采用	cǎi-yòng	select	13.5
菜	cài	vegetables	7.5
参考	cān-kǎo	consult	9.8
残废	cán-fèi	permanent disablement	12.4
残霤	cán-liù	cracked gutter	11.6
苍白	cāng-bái	greenish white	8.4
藏	cáng	store	1.3
糙	cāo	coarse	6.6
嘈杂	cáo-zá	noisy	13.4
侧	cè	side	1.3
曾	céng	once; before	4.3
层	céng	layer	10.3
差别	chā-bié	difference	7.2
茶叶	chá-yè	tea leaves	7.5
察	chá	examine; investigate	10.8
察色	chá-sè	inspect a color	10.2
察舌	chá-shé	inspection of the tongue	10.3
柴胡	chái-hú	(drug name) Bupleurum chi-nense D C.	3.7
缠喉症	chán-hóu-zhèng	pathocondition of "strangled throat"	13.2
蟾酥	chán-sū	toad venom	15.2
产	chǎn	deliver; delivery	5.4
产地	chǎn-dì	place of production; place of origin	16.1
产生	chǎn-shēng	produce	5.3
产物	chǎn-wù	product	15.8
场所	chǎng-suǒ	location	14.3
尝试	cháng-shì	test; taste	16.6
常	cháng	often; regular	3.5
常常	cháng-cháng	often; regularly	2.8

常法	cháng-fǎ	common pattern	12.5
常见	cháng-jiàn	often	5.3
常气	cháng-qì	normal qi	6.1
常数	cháng-shù	constant; regularly	11.3
常用	cháng-yòng	employ often	4.3
长	cháng	extended (pulse condition)	11.2
长期	cháng-qī	longtime	3.8
长时期	cháng-shí-qī	long-term	3.4
长途	cháng-tú	long way; long distance	6.4
长夏	cháng-xià	late summer	2.5
肠	cháng	intestine	1.5
肠鸣	cháng-míng	intestinal sounds	6.3
肠胃病	cháng-wèi-bìng	illnesses of the intestines and of the stomach	7.4
畅	chàng	unimpeded; unconstrained	10.6
潮	cháo	moist	1.5
潮	cháo	wave	8.4
潮热	cháo-rè	tidal fever	8.4
潮湿	cháo-shī	moisture	6.5
炒	chǎo	fry	16.2
彻底	chè-dǐ	carefully	1.8
臣	chén	minister	14.1
臣药	chén-yào	minister drug	14.2
沉	chén	deep	1.5
沉寒	chén-hán	deep-seated cold	13.6
沉极	chén-jí	extremely deep (pulse condition)	11.5
称	chēng	designate; call	4.4
称号	chēng-hào	title; designation	4.2
称为	chēng-wéi	call	4.1
称做 (作)	chēng-zuò	be called; call	1.7
成	chéng	constitute	1.2

成	chéng	become; form	5.8
成方	chéng-fāng	established prescription	5.6
成熟	chéng-shú	maturing	16.1
成为	chéng-wéi	constitute	1.1
成形	chéng-xíng	assume physical shape	13.7
成药	chéng-yào	ready-made medication	15.5
成竹	chéng-zhú	the complete bamboo (a metaphor taken from painting, indicating a well-thought-out plan)	15.7
呈	chéng	manifest; present	5.5
呈现	chéng-xiàn	bring forth	6.3
乘	chéng	seize, exploit (a weakness), take advantage	2.4
程度	chéng-dù	degree	7.7
程序	chéng-xù	sequence; order	9.6
承受	chéng-shòu	take in; receive	4.6
痴	chī	idiocy	7.1
迟	chí	retarded; slow	1.5
迟钝	chí-dùn	retarded	12.2
齿	chǐ	tooth	3.6
齿痛	chǐ-tòng	toothache	3.6
尺	chǐ	foot	11.1
赤	chì	red	2.5
充	chōng	complete	5.6
充斥	chōng-chì	fill	6.7
充实	chōng-shí	abundant	2.4
冲服	chōng-fú	take in (with a liquid)	15.3
虫	chóng	worm	7.5
虫兽伤	chóng-shòu shāng	injury from insects and animals	7.7
重	chóng	doubled	1.6
重复	chóng-fù	repeat; repetitive	14.7
重寒	chóng-hán	doubled cold	1.6

重热	chóng-rè	doubled heat	1.6
冲	chòng	penetrate	9.4
稠厚	chóu-hòu	thick	15.3
臭	chòu	fetid	10.7
臭秽	chòu-huì	foul	8.5
初	chū	just before	10.4
初步	chū-bù	preliminary	3.8
初期	chū-qī	initial phase	9.2
初起	chū-qǐ	begin	6.4
出	chū	leave	10.7
出发	chū-fā	proceed from	12.1
出来	chū-lái	lit.: come out (particle indicating the outcome of a process indicated by the immediately preceding verb)	1.2
出纳	chū-nà	putting out and taking in; input and output	4.1
出入	chū-rù	difference	14.8
出生	chū-shēng	be born; give birth	5.5
出现	chū-xiàn	let appear; bring forth	4.2
出血	chū-xuè	hemorrhage	5.4
出血不止	chū-xuè-bù-zhǐ	incessant bleeding	5.3
出于	chū-yú	leave from	5.7
除	chú	eliminate	12.3
除...外	chú ... wài	except for ...	8.4
除此以外	chú-cǐ-yǐ-wài	in addition	14.7
除了	chú-le	except for	7.3
除去不用	chú-qù-bú-yòng	omit altogether	14.8
除去	chú-qù	discard	16.2
处方	chǔ-fāng	prescription; write a prescription	3.6
处理	chǔ-lǐ	deal with; sort out; handle	2.8
触	chù	strike; rise to	10.7

触按	chù-àn	touch	11.7
触诊	chù-zhěn	examination through touching (the patient)	11.1
处	chù	locality	1.3
川贝母	chuān-bèi-mǔ	(the drug) beimu from (the province of Si)chuan	16.1
川桂枝	chuān-guì-zhī	(the drug) guizhi from (the province of Si)chuan	16.1
川黄柏	chuān-huáng-bò	(the drug) huangbo from (the province of Si)chuan	16.1
川芎	chuān-xiōng	(drug name) Ligusticum wallichii Franch.	16.1
传	chuán	transmit	3.2
传	chuán	transmit; be transmitted	8.3
传变	chuán-biàn	transmission and transformation	3.5
传导	chuán-dǎo	transmit; transmission	1.3
传化	chuán-huà	transmit and transform	4.1
传经	chuán-jīng	conduit-transmission	9.5
传染	chuán-rǎn	infection through transmission	6.8
传入	chuán-rù	transmit into	9.6
传尸痨	chuán-shī-láo	consumption transmitted by corpses	7.5
喘	chuǎn	pant	14.3
喘喝	chuǎn-hè	pant	6.4
喘息	chuǎn-xī	pant	7.3
创口	chuāng-kǒu	opening of a wound	7.7
创伤	chuāng-shāng	wound	5.4
创立	chuàng-lì	establish; found	1.2
春	chūn	spring	2.5
唇	chún	lip	6.6
纯实	chún-shí	pure repletion	8.6
纯虚	chún-xū	pure depletion	8.6
慈葱	cí-cōng	tender spring onion	11.2

此	cǐ	this	2.1
此时	cǐ-shí	at this time	9.2
此外	cǐ-wài	furthermore	1.7
刺	cì	prick	3.6
刺激	cì-jī	stimulus	4.2
次	cì	-times	15.3
次序	cì-xù	sequence	2.5
次要	cì-yào	of secondary importance	12.5
次于	cì yú	be secondary to	16.5
从	cóng	from	1.3
从 ... 内	cóng ... nèi	from within	5.1
从 ... 入手	cóng ... rù-shǒu	start from ...	11.3
从 ... 上	cóng ... shàng	starting from ...; on the basis of	2.8
从 ... 中	cóng ... zhōng	from ...	2.1
从 A 来说	cóng A lái shuo	lit: "from (the point of view of) A;" as far as A is concerned	8.5
从而	cóng-ér	hence; therefore	1.1
从属	cóng-shǔ	categorize	2.5
凑	còu	hit	11.6
腠理	còu-lǐ	porous structures	5.7
粗	cū	rough	10.6
醋	cù	vinegar	16.3
醋制	cù-zhì	processing with vinegar	16.3
促	cù	hasty (pulse condition)	11.2
促进	cù-jìn	stimulate	16.8
促使	cù-shǐ	lead to	12.7
猝然	cù-rán	sudden	6.2
窜入	cuàn-rù	enter; invade	9.6
催吐	cuī-tù	induced vomiting	13.1
催吐药	cuī-tù-yào	drugs inducing vomiting; emetic drugs	13.2
存在	cún-zài	be present; exist	1.2

寸	cùn	inch	11.1
寸白虫	cùn-bái-chóng	tapeworm	7.5
寸口	cùn-kǒu	inch opening	11.1
撮空	cuō-kōng	grasp into the empty (air)	10.5
措	cuò	make use of	12.6
措施	cuò-shī	measure; approach	12.4
错乱	cuò-luàn	uncontrolled	7.1
错杂	cuò-zá	mixed	8.6
错综	cuò-zōng	complicated	3.1
错综复杂	cuò-zōng-fù-zá	complex	8.1

D

达	dá	reach	16.8
达到...以后	dá-dào ... yǐ-hòu	after ... has been attained	12.7
达到	dá-dào	attain; reach	12.7
大	dà	big; major	5.1
大便	dà-biàn	stool	4.3
大肠	dà-cháng	large intestine	4.1
大承气汤	dà-chéng-qì-tāng	large formula to contain the qi	14.5
大多	dà-duō	mostly; in general	3.5
大方	dà-fāng	large formula	14.5
大概	dà-gài	as a rule; most likely	15.7
大汗	dà-hàn	major sweating	14.5
大家	dà-jiā	all; everybody	3.6
大体上	dà-tǐ-shàng	in general	15.6
大丸	dà-wán	large pills	15.1
大下	dà-xià	major purgation	14.5

大小	dà-xiǎo	size; age	6.8
大约	dà-yuē	in general	15.1
带	dài	carry along	10.7
带来	dài-lái	cause; lead to	12.4
带粘性	dài-nián-xìng	sticky	15.2
带下病	dài-xià-bìng	illness below the belt; gynecological illness	10.2
代	dài	intermittent (pulse condition)	11.2
代表	dài-biǎo	represent	1.2
代名词	dài-míng-cí	synonym	1.8
待	dài	wait	5.5
待到 ... 以后	dài-dào ... yǐ-hòu	after ...	5.5
丹	dān	pellet; (a pellet-sized or powder preparation, sometimes produced by means of chemical processes)	15.1
丹剂	dān-jì	pellet preparation	15.3
单	dān	only	5.6
单按	dān-àn	feel with one (finger)	11.1
单独	dān-dú	individually	15.5
单数	dān-shù	odd numbers	14.6
单味	dān-wèi	single drugs	14.1
单味药	dān-wèi-yào	single substance drug	14.4
胆	dǎn	gallbladder	4.1
胆火	dǎn-huǒ	fire of the gallbladder	4.5
旦夕	dàn-xī	dawn and dusk; in one day	12.8
但	dàn	but	1.8
但是	dàn-shì	however; but	5.6
啖	dàn	eat	6.4
淡	dàn	pale	1.5
淡黄	dàn-huáng	pale yellow	10.4
淡渗	dàn-shèn	bland seeping	13.7

弹	dàn	round	11.5
弹丸	dàn-wán	bullet	15.1
当	dāng	should; must	1.8
当 ... 时	dāng ... shí	at the time when ...	2.6
当然	dāng-rán	of course	5.4
党参	dǎng-shēn	(drug name) Codonopsis pilosula (Franch.) Nannf.	16.1
荡	dàng	sweep away	13.7
刀剑	dāo-jiàn	knives and swords	7.7
刀伤	dāo-shāng	injury from a knife	7.7
倒仆	dǎo-pū	collapse	6.2
导	dǎo	guide	13.7
导下	dǎo-xià	guide downwards	13.7
导致	dǎo-zhì	lead to	12.1
到	dào	to; with	2.6
到达	dào-dá	reach	15.1
道	dào	Way; doctrine; principle	11.8
道理	dào-lǐ	principle	1.2
盗汗	dào-hàn	thief sweating	7.5
得	dé	receive	5.4
得出	dé-chū	get	8.1
的	de	(particle defining a possessive)	1.1
的	de	(particle defining the immediately preceding expression as a state of being)	1.1
地	de	(particle defining the immediately preceding expression as an adverb; roughly equivalent to the English "..ly")	1.1
等	děng	(particle defining the end of an enumeration)	1.1
等	... děng	... and so on; such as ...	4.6
等等	děng-děng	and so on	2.6

等量	děng-liàng	equal amount	15.2
等于	děng-yú	be comparable to	5.7
低	dī	deep	10.6
低怯	dī-qiè	faint	4.3
滴	dī	drop	11.6
涤痰	dí-tán	flush away phlegm	13.7
抵触	dǐ-chù	be in conflict	14.4
地	dì	soil	6.4
地步	dì-bù	condition; stage	12.7
地方	dì-fāng	location, place	5.2
地黄	dì-huáng	(drug name) Rhemannia glutinosa (Gaertn.) Libosch.	1.7
地位	dì-wèi	position	7.3
第	dì	(particle indicating that the following number is an ordinal number)	8.1
第二次	dì-èr-cì	the second time	15.5
第一次	dì-yī-cì	the first time	15.5
颠倒	diān-dǎo	confusion	6.7
癫	diān	insanity	7.1
癫狂	diān-kuáng	mania and/or depression	10.6
点	diǎn	spot	7.5
跌打	diē-dǎ	fall	7.7
锭剂	dìng-jì	ingot preparation	15.3
定	dìng	fix	11.6
定出	dìng-chū	decide	8.8
定名	dìng-míng	name	11.1
定义	dìng-yì	define	10.3
定志	dìng-zhì	stabilize the will	5.6
东	dōng	east	2.5
冬	dōng	winter	2.5
冬季	dōng-jì	winter	15.3

冬天	dōng-tiān	winter	6.8
懂得	dǒng-de	understand	8.1
动	dòng	move; movement	1.3
动脉	dòng-mài	pulsating vessel	11.1
动态	dòng-tài	nature of movement	1.5
动作	dòng-zuò	movement	10.5
都	dōu	all	1.2
都是	dōu-shì	always; all; in each case	1.8
斗争	dòu-zhēng	fight	10.1
豆	dòu	bean	11.3
豆浆	dòu-jiāng	soy-bean milk	10.4
豆蔻	dòu-kòu	(drug name) Amomum cardamomum L.	1.7
毒厉	dú-lì	pernicious	6.8
毒热	dú-rè	poison heat	10.5
毒蛇	dú-shé	poisonous snake	7.7
毒性	dú-xìng	toxicity	14.1
独	dú	alone; only	10.2
独立	dú-lì	independent	4.1
渎	dú	ditch	4.7
堵塞	dǔ-sè	block	13.2
度	dù	degree	15.3
端	duān	end; point; (measure word)	10.2
短	duǎn	short; (in the present context in conjunction with the character niao [urine]:) scant urine	6.6
断绝	duàn-jué	stop; break off	10.6
对	duì	on; at	3.8
对比	duì-bǐ	balance; comparison	9.5
对称	duì-chèn	symmetrical	4.8
对待	duì-dài	treat	5.2
对立	duì-lì	antagonistic	1.2

对象	duì-xiàng	target	13.6
对于	duì-yú	on	4.3
顿	dùn	suddenly	11.6
多	duō	many; often	1.4
多少	duō-shǎo	many and few; amount	14.5
多数	duō-shù	mostly; often	5.3

E

恶	è	bad	13.2
恶化	è-huà	aggravate; aggravation	12.7
恶劣	è-liè	vile; foul	16.2
而	ér	and; and yet	1.2
而已	ér-yǐ	lit.: "and thereby ending" (particle indicating the close of an argument: "that's it"; often used in the sense of: "and nothing else"; "that's all")	12.1
耳	ěr	ear	2.6
耳鸣	ěr-míng	ringing in the ears	4.4
二	èr	two	9.2
二百	èr-bǎi	two hundred	15.1
二便	èr-biàn	stools and urine	10.6
二陈汤	èr-chén-tāng	decoction with two old (drugs)	14.7
二煎	èr-jiān	the second boiling	15.5
二十八	èr-shí-bā	twenty eight	11.2
二者	èr-zhě	both	5.2

F

发	fā	develop; appear	1.4
发	fā	develop; bring forth	6.5
发斑	fā-bān	develop macules	6.7
发病	fā-bìng	breakout of an illness	1.4
发汗	fā-hàn	develop sweat	8.6
发汗法	fā-hàn-fǎ	(therapeutic) pattern inducing perspiration	1.8
发挥	fā-huī	elaborate	14.4
发热	fā-rè	develop a fever; fever	1.4
发散	fā-sàn	disperse	16.3
发生	fā-shēng	develop; generate	3.5
发现	fā-xiàn	find; discover	1.2
发育	fā-yù	development	5.5
发展	fā-zhǎn	development	8.8
发疹	fā-zhěn	develop pustules	6.7
乏力	fá-lì	lack of physical strength	8.5
法	fǎ	(therapeutic) pattern	1.6
法度	fǎ-dù	law	14.1
法则	fǎ-zé	rule; law	12.3
番	fān	(measure word for activities)	9.8
凡	fán	all	4.1
凡是	fán-shì	all; whenever	1.4
烦闷	fán-mèn	uneasiness and chest pressure	5.6
烦躁	fán-zào	vexation	6.7
燔灼	fán-zhuó	burn	6.7
反	fǎn	opposite	1.2
反常	fǎn-cháng	unusual	2.4
反复	fǎn-fù	return; repeat	9.3
反过来	fǎn-guò-lái	conversely	2.4

反来	fǎn-lái	conversely; on the contrary	2.4
反映	fǎn-yìng	appear; be reflected in	3.5
反应	fǎn-yìng	reaction	14.1
反之	fǎn-zhī	in contrast	8.5
反治	fǎn-zhì	paradoxical treatment	12.1
反治法	fǎn-zhì-fǎ	paradox therapy pattern	12.3
范畴	fàn-chóu	realm; category	3.8
范围	fàn-wéi	spectrum	6.6
犯	fàn	offend	2.7
泛滥	fàn-làn	inundation	12.7
芳	fāng	aromatic	13.4
芳化	fāng-huà	transform (dampness) by means of fragrant (drugs)	13.4
芳香	fāng-xiāng	fragrant; aromatic	1.7
方	fāng	prescription	9.8
方案	fāng-àn	program	15.8
方才	fāng-cái	then	6.8
方法	fāng-fǎ	method	1.1
方剂	fāng-jì	formula	13.5
方面	fāng-miàn	aspect	1.1
...方面	... fāng-miàn	as for ...	6.1
方位	fāng-wèi	position; cardinal point	2.5
方向	fāng-xiàng	orientation	12.2
方针	fāng-zhēn	approach	8.8
方制	fāng-zhì	system of prescribing	14.1
房室	fáng-shì	bedroom	7.7
房室伤	fáng-shì-shāng	harm from sexual intercourse	7.7
防	fáng	prevent	10.1
防止	fáng-zhǐ	prevent	2.7
放	fàng	let	15.4
非	fēi	be not	4.8
非 ... 不可	fēi ... bù-kě	impossible if not ...	8.8

非 ... 不 ...	fēi ... bù ...	only if ... is ...	4.5
非但 ... 而且	fēi-dàn ... ér-qiě	not only ..., but also	2.8
肥	féi	fat	7.5
肺	fèi	lung	2.6
肺风	fèi-fēng	lung wind	10.5
肺绝	fèi-jué	lung failure	10.5
肺劳	fèi-láo	taxation of the lung	2.8
肺气	fèi-qì	lung qi	4.3
肺热	fèi-rè	lung heat	7.3
肺热病	fèi-rè-bìng	lung heat illness	10.2
肺痈	fèi-yōng	lung abscess	10.7
肺脏	fèi-zàng	lung	4.3
沸	fèi	boil; seethe	11.6
分	fēn	differentiate; order	1.3
分辨	fēn-biàn	differentiate	8.3
分别	fēn-bié	differentiate	1.7
分不出	fēn-bù-chū	impossible to distinguish	15.7
分部	fēn-bù	individual regions	10.3
分开	fēn-kāi	separate; separately	15.5
分类	fēn-lèi	categorize	9.8
分离	fēn-lí	separate	4.8
分配	fēn-pèi	associate separately with	10.2
分属	fēn-shǔ	assign	3.6
分为	fēn-wéi	divide into	3.2
分析	fēn-xī	analyze	2.6
分研	fēn-yán	grind separately	15.2
分有	fēn-yǒu	distinguish	1.5
分作	fēn-zuò	categorize	1.4
粉	fěn	powder	15.1
粉剂	fěn-jì	pulverized preparation	15.2
分	fèn	section	5.3

丰	fēng	rich	16.1
丰富	fēng-fù	rich	15.8
风	fēng	wind	1.8
风寒	fēng-hán	wind cold	3.7
风火	fēng-huǒ	wind-fire	6.2
风热	fēng-rè	wind-heat	6.2
风湿	fēng-shī	wind-dampness	6.2
风暑	fēng-shǔ	wind-summerheat	6.2
风痰	fēng-tán	wind-phlegm	7.3
风温	fēng-wēn	wind-warmth	6.2
风邪	fēng-xié	wind evil	6.1
风燥	fēng-zào	wind-dryness	6.2
蜂蜜制	fēng-mì-zhì	processing with honey	16.3
否	fǒu	no; not	9.5
否认	fǒu-rèn	deny	14.4
否则	fǒu-zé	if not then; otherwise	2.3
扶	fú	support	12.5
扶持	fú-chí	support	12.1
扶阳	fú-yáng	support the yang	13.6
扶正	fú-zhèng	support the proper	12.5
符	fú	belong together	11.8
符合	fú-hé	be in keeping with; coincide	11.4
伏	fú	hide	6.3
伏邪	fú-xié	hidden evil	6.8
伏饮	fú-yǐn	hidden drinks	11.4
服	fú	consume	15.5
服法	fú-fǎ	mode of intake	15.5
服食	fú-shí	consume; take in (a medication)	15.1
服药	fú-yào	take drugs	13.2
服用	fú-yòng	consume	15.3
浮	fú	at the surface	1.5

338

浮	fú	bloated	6.5
浮浮泛泛	fú-fú-fàn-fàn	float or bob at the surface; superficial and volatile (intensification of meaning through doubling)	11.6
浮极	fú-jí	extremely superficial (pulse condition)	11.5
浮躁	fú-zào	impatient	11.8
浮肿	fú-zhǒng	edema	4.3
跗	fú	instep	11.7
辅助药	fǔ-zhù-yào	helper drug	14.3
俯	fǔ	bent	10.5
俯仰	fǔ-yǎng	lower or lift (the head)	5.6
釜沸	fǔ-fèi	seething cauldron (pulse condition)	11.6
府	fǔ	palace	4.6
腐	fǔ	putrid	10.7
腐败	fǔ-bài	decay; rot	6.8
腐熟	fǔ-shú	decompose	4.6
副作用	fù-zuò-yòng	side effect	16.8
复	fù	return	12.5
复方	fù-fāng	compound formula	14.5
复来	fù-lái	return	11.6
复杂	fù-zá	complex; complicated	7.3
腹	fù	abdomen	7.4
腹部	fù-bù	abdominal section	12.7
腹满	fù-mǎn	abdominal fullness	6.5
腹水	fù-shuǐ	abdominal water	12.7
腹痛	fù-tòng	abdominal pain	6.3
腹泻	fù-xiè	diarrhea	14.6
腹胀	fù-zhàng	abdominal swelling	8.2
负责	fù-zé	be responsible for (something)	4.6

附子	fù-zǐ	(drug name) Aconitum carmi-chaeli Debx.	1.7
妇	fù	woman	3.8
妇女	fù-nǚ	woman	10.2
妇人	fù-rén	woman	5.4

G

改	gǎi	change	15.7
改变	gǎi-biàn	change	7.2
改善	gǎi-shàn	improve	5.2
改为	gǎi-wéi	replace by	14.8
概	gài	in general; summarily	8.3
概况	gài-kuàng	rough survey	8.3
概括	gài-kuò	outline	16.5
概括地说	gài-kuò-de-shuō	generally speaking; to put it briefly	1.4
概括性	gài-kuò-xìng	general	1.8
干	gān	dry	5.8
干姜	gān-jiāng	(drug name) dried ginger	1.7
干咳	gān-ké	dry coughing	6.6
干燥	gān-zào	dryness	6.6
甘	gān	sweet	1.7
甘草	gān-cǎo	(drug name) Glycyrrhiza uralensis Fisch.	14.8
甘凉剂	gān-liáng-jì	sweet and cooling formula	6.6
甘味	gān-wèi	sweet flavor	16.6
竿	gān	cane	11.3
肝	gān	liver	1.7

340

肝病	gān-bìng	liver illness	2.7
肝风	gān-fēng	liver wind	10.5
肝火	gān-huǒ	liver fire	1.8
肝火上逆	gān-huǒ-shàng-nì	adversely rising liver fire	10.2
肝气	gān-qì	liver qi	2.7
肝热病	gān-rè-bìng	liver heat illness	10.2
肝旺	gān-wàng	liver effulgence	2.7
肝虚	gān-xū	liver depletion	2.7
肝阳	gān-yáng	liver yang	13.5
肝脏	gān-zàng	liver	4.2
疳积	gān-jī	malnutrition accumulation	7.5
感	gǎn	be affected	6.4
感冒	gǎn-mào	common cold	1.8
感染	gǎn-rǎn	affect; be affected by	6.2
感受	gǎn-shòu	be affected	6.4
刚强	gāng-qiáng	strength	4.2
肛门	gāng-mén	anus	7.5
纲领	gāng-lǐng	guiding principle	8.1
纲要	gāng-yào	fundamental categories	1.5
高	gāo	high	10.1
高低	gāo-dī	high and low; level	10.6
高骨	gāo-gǔ	elevated bone	11.1
高级	gāo-jí	high-level	5.6
膏	gāo	paste	15.1
膏剂	gāo-jì	paste preparations	15.3
膏粱	gāo-liáng	rich food	6.5
膏药	gāo-yào	paste drug	15.3
膏滋药	gāo-zī-yào	pasty nutritious drug	15.3
革	gé	tympanic (pulse condition)	11.2
葛根	gé-gēn	(drug name) Pueraria lobata (Willd.) Ohwi.	3.7

格阳于外	gé-yáng-yú-wài	repelled yang (i.e., misleading heat in the outside in case of severe cold in the interior of the body)	12.2
格阻	gé-zǔ	barricade	12.2
膈	gé	diaphragm	5.3
隔	gé	distance; separation	2.8
个人	gè-rén	each person	10.8
各个	gè-ge	each	1.1
个	ge	(general measure word)	1.2
根本	gēn-běn	basic root	12.5
根据	gēn-jù	on the basis of; in accordancc with; basis	1.4
根源	gēn-yuán	basic source	12.5
跟着	gēn-zhe	following	6.2
更	gèng	even more; further	2.3
更...一步	gèng ... yī-bù	even more ...	9.4
更好	gèng-hǎo	better	16.8
工作	gōng-zuò	work; activity	2.7
攻	gōng	attack	8.6
攻下	gōng-xià	offensive purgation	13.1
攻下剂	gōng-xià-jì	remedies for a charge downwards	13.3
攻阵	gōng-zhèn	attacking array	14.7
功	gōng	success	13.7
功夫	gōng-fū	effort; work	9.8
功能	gōng-néng	function	1.3
功效	gōng-xiào	efficacy	16.1
共	gòng	together	11.1
狗脊	gǒu-jǐ	(drug name) Cibotium barometz (L.) J. Sm.	3.7
垢	gòu	staining	10.3
构成	gòu-chéng	constitute	1.1

孤立	gū-lì	isolate	2.8
鼓	gǔ	drum	11.7
鼓皮	gǔ-pí	drum skin	11.2
古	gǔ	old; antiquity	1.2
古人	gǔ-rén	people of antiquity; the ancients	1.2
古为今用	gǔ wéi jīn yòng	make the old useful for today	14.4
骨	gǔ	bone	1.3
骨病	gǔ-bìng	bone illness	10.5
骨节痛	gǔ-jié-tòng	bone and joint pain	13.1
骨蒸	gǔ-zhēng	steaming bones	7.5
故	gù	hence; therefore	1.3
顾	gù	observe	7.3
固定	gù-dìng	identify definitely	14.8
固精	gù-jīng	stabilize semen	12.5
固涩	gù-sè	contract; (application of) astringent (remedies)	4.6
固阵	gù-zhèn	consolidating array	14.7
固执	gù-zhí	stubbornly cling to (something)	6.3
痼冷	gù-lěng	obstinate frigidity	11.4
瓜果	guā-guǒ	gourds	6.4
怪	guài	uncommon	11.6
关	guān	affect; concern	10.4
关	guān	pass gate	11.1
关键	guān-jiàn	key point	8.1
关键性	guān-jiàn-xìng	central; essential	12.3
关节	guān-jié	joint	3.1
关系	guān-xi	relationship	1.2
关于	guān-yú	as regards	8.1
官	guān	official	4.7
观察	guān-chá	observe	1.2
贯串	guàn-chuàn	permeate; penetrate	1.1
光	guāng	shine	10.4

光舌	guāng-shé	shiny tongue	10.4
广	guǎng	wide	6.2
广泛	guǎng-fàn	extensive; comprehensive	1.8
广木香	guǎng-mù-xiāng	(the drug) muxiang from (the province of) Guang(dong)	16.1
广义	guǎng-yì	broad sense	5.5
规律	guī-lǜ	law	9.8
归	guī	identify as	1.4
归经	guī-jīng	conduit entry	16.7
归类	guī-lèi	categorize; classify	2.6
归纳	guī-nà	draw inductive conclusions	1.2
归入	guī-rù	associate with	16.7
归属	guī-shǔ	belong	4.1
归于	guī-yú	turn to	4.6
归于	guī-yú	associate with	5.5
轨	guǐ	track; rails	6.1
桂枝	guì-zhī	(drug name) Cinnamomum cassia Blume	14.2
桂枝汤	guì-zhī-tāng	decoction with guizhi	14.7
贵重	guì-zhòng	expensive	15.2
腘	guó	popliteal fossa	3.5
过	guò	excessive; too much	6.5
过	guò	(particle indicating the conclusion of the process expressed by the immediately preceding verb)	14.4
过程	guò-chéng	process	2.5
过度	guò-dù	excessive	5.4
过多	guò-duō	too much	5.4
过滤	guò-lǜ	filtrate	15.3
过去	guò-qù	earlier; formerly	15.7
过一个时期	guò-yī-ge-shí-qī	after a (certain) time	15.4

H

孩儿茶	hái-ér-chá	catechu; (drug name) Acacia katechu (L.) Willd.	15.2
还	hái	still; in addition	2.4
还	hái	also; in addition	5.3
还是	hái-shì	still	16.1
还有	hái-yǒu	there is yet another ...	2.4
海	hǎi	sea	4.5
含有	hán-yǒu	include	1.6
寒	hán	cold	1.4
寒病	hán-bìng	cold illness	16.4
寒凉	hán-liáng	cold	5.4
寒凉药	hán-liáng-yào	cold-cool drug	16.5
寒湿	hán-shī	cold damp	11.4
寒痰	hán-tán	cold-phlegm	7.3
寒象	hán-xiàng	cold signs	1.6
寒邪	hán-xié	cold evil	5.4
寒性	hán-xìng	cold nature	1.4
寒性病	hán-xìng-bìng	illnesses of a cold nature	13.6
寒性药	hán-xìng-yào	drug of cold nature	16.4
寒药	hán-yào	cold drugs	12.2
寒疫	hán-yì	cold epidemics	6.8
寒阵	hán-zhèn	cooling array	14.7
寒症	hán-zhèng	pathoconditions of cold	1.4
汗	hàn	sweat; perspiration	1.6
汗出	hàn-chū	sweat	5.7
汗法	hàn-fǎ	(therapeutic) pattern inducing perspiration	1.6
汉朝	hàn-cháo	the Han dynasty (206 BCE to 221 CE)	14.4

行	háng	column	15.7
好	hǎo	(particle indicating the conclusion of the activity or process signified by the immediately preceding verb)	15.6
好	hǎo	good	16.8
好处	hǎo-chù	benefit; advantage	15.8
好些	hǎo-xiē	many	3.8
耗散	hào-sàn	dispersion	12.2
皓白	hào-bái	shiny white	7.5
和	hé	with; and	2.7
和	hé	and	1.1
和	hé	balanced	11.3
和 ... 一样	hé ... yī-yàng	in the same way as ...	2.7
和法	hé-fǎ	the pattern of harmonization	13.4
和肝	hé-gān	harmonize the liver	12.7
和缓	hé-huǎn	mild	13.4
和解	hé-jiě	harmonization and resolution	13.1
和解法	hé-jiě-fǎ	pattern of reconciliation	13.4
和平	hé-píng	balanced	13.8
和阵	hé-zhèn	harmonizing array	14.7
和中方法	hé-zhōng-fāng-fǎ	pattern to harmonize the center	13.2
合	hé	together	10.3
合病	hé-bìng	parallel illnesses	9.7
合并	hé-bìng	combine	15.3
合谷	hé-gǔ	the he-gu (hole)	3.6
合乎	hé-hū	conform	1.1
合理	hé-lǐ	be appropriate	12.6
合适	hé-shì	appropriate	16.7
合研	hé-yán	grind together	15.2
合作	hé-zuò	cooperation	3.8
涸	hé	dry up	13.3

346

黑	hēi	black	2.5
黑豆	hēi-dòu	black soybean	16.3
很	hěn	very	5.3
横	héng	crosswise	3.1
洪	hóng	vast	6.4
洪水	hóng-shuǐ	flood; flood water	12.7
红	hóng	red; reddening	1.4
红汗	hóng-hàn	"red sweat" (i.e., nosebleeding)	5.7
喉	hóu	throat	6.7
喉症	hóu-zhèng	pathoconditions (affecting) the throat	13.2
厚	hòu	thick; rich in contents	6.5
候	hòu	examine	11.1
候	hòu	sign	11.6
候测	hòu-cè	assess	11.1
后	hòu	after	2.6
后	hòu	back; behind	3.3
后病	hòu-bìng	the later illness	12.8
后来	hòu-lái	later one	14.4
后脑	hòu-nǎo	metencephalon	3.7
后人	hòu-rén	people in later times	12.3
后天	hòu-tiān	the later dependence	4.3
后遗症	hòu-yí-zhèng	sequelae (of an illness)	12.4
呼	hū	call	7.5
呼吸	hū-xī	breath	8.5
忽然	hū-rán	all of a sudden	12.8
忽视	hū-shì	neglect; ignore	12.6
琥珀	hǔ-pò	amber	5.6
互	hù	mutual	13.6
互相	hù-xiāng	each other	3.3
花	huā	flower	15.8
滑	huá	smooth	1.5

滑精	huá-jīng	involuntary seminal efflux	4.4
滑泄	huá xiè	efflux diarrhea	14.7
化	huà	transform	1.3
化出	huà-chū	derive by modification	11.2
化脓性	huà-nóng-xìng	suppurating	1.8
化痰	huà-tán	transform phlegm	12.5
环	huán	circle	3.3
环	huán	link (in a chain)	10.3
环境	huán-jìng	environment	5.2
缓	huǎn	relaxed	9.2
缓补	huǎn-bǔ	mild supplementation	13.8
缓方	huǎn-fāng	mild formula	14.5
缓和	huǎn-hé	alleviate	12.6
缓缓	huǎn-huǎn	mildly	13.8
缓下	huǎn-xià	mild purging	13.3
患	huàn	suffer (from an illness)	5.5
涣散	huàn-sàn	slacken	5.6
黄	huáng	yellow	1.5
黄疸	huáng-dǎn	jaundice	10.2
黄连	huáng-lián	(drug name) Coptis chinensis Franch.	1.7
恍惚	huǎng-hū	absentminded	7.1
灰黑	huī-hēi	gray-black	10.4
挥发性	huī-fā-xìng	volatile	15.2
恢复	huī-fù	recovery	5.3
蛔虫	huí-chóng	roundworm	7.5
回	huí	return	11.3
回阳	huí-yáng	have the yang return	6.3
回转	huí-zhuǎn	return	5.8
秽	huì	filth; dirty matter	6.8
会	huì	can; be able to	3.5
昏	hūn	confused	3.5

昏迷	hūn-mí	confusion	4.2
浑身	hún-shēn	the entire body	12.6
浑浊	hún-zhuó	turbid	10.7
混合	hùn-hé	mix	15.2
混同	hùn-tóng	mixed	9.4
混为一谈	hùn-wéi-yī-tán	speak of separate entities as a single entity; confuse	5.5
豁痰	huō-tán	clear away phlegm	13.7
活动	huó-dòng	activity	3.4
活络	huó-luò	activate the network (vessels)	15.4
活泼	huó-po	active	5.6
火	huǒ	fire	1.2
火亢	huǒ-kàng	hyperactivity of fire	10.2
火气	huǒ-qì	fire qi	4.2
火灼烧伤	huǒ-zhuó-shāo-shāng	burn	7.7
或	huò	or	1.5
或者	huò-zhě	or if	14.3
豁豁然	huò-huò-rán	fragile; breakable	11.2

J

基本	jī-běn	basic	1.1
基础	jī-chǔ	basis	5.5
基于	jī-yú	be based on	10.1
机动	jī-dòng	adaptation; flexible; expedient	1.8
机会	jī-huì	opportunity	9.5
机能	jī-néng	function	1.4
机转	jī-zhuǎn	process	8.5
积	jī	accumulate	6.4

积极	jī-jí	positive	4.4
积聚	jī-jù	conglomeration	13.7
积热	jī-rè	heat accumulation	10.7
积弱	jī-ruò	very weak	13.8
积食	jī-shí	food accumulation	13.2
积滞	jī-zhì	accumulation blockages	13.3
肌	jī	muscle	1.3
肌表	jī-biǎo	muscular exterior	13.1
肌肤	jī-fū	the (human) skin	3.5
肌肉	jī-ròu	muscles	8.2
肌肉消瘦	jī-ròu-xiāo-shòu	emaciation	4.3
饥	jī	be hungry; hunger	6.6
鸡毛	jī-máo	a chicken's feather	13.2
奇方	jī-fāng	unpaired formula	14.5
极	jí	extreme	6.1
极大	jí-dà	very big	7.2
极度	jí-dù	extreme	11.6
极端	jí-duān	extreme	16.5
极其	jí-qí	extremely	2.8
极速	jí-sù	very fast	6.8
极小丸	jí-xiǎo-wán	extremely small pill	15.1
极虚	jí-xū	extreme depletion	13.8
及	jí	reach	2.4
及	jí	and	3.7
及时	jí-shí	in due time	9.2
急方	jí-fāng	urgent formula	14.5
急惊	jí-jīng	acute fright	10.2
急切	jí-qiè	fast	14.5
急躁	jí-zào	rashness and impatience	4.5
急症	jí-zhèng	critical pathocondition	10.1
疾	jí	hurried (pulse condition)	11.2

疾病	jí-bìng	illness	3.5
即	jí	namely; that is	1.4
即	jí	immediately	6.8
即使 ... 也不 ...	jí shǐ ... yě bù ...	even if ... nevertheless not ...	7.2
几	jǐ	some	7.8
几个	jǐ-gè	some	7.8
几十	jǐ-shí	tens of	14.1
给养	jǐ-yǎng	nourishment	5.5
给予	jǐ-yǔ	provide	12.2
季节	jì-jié	season	2.5
剂	jì	formula	6.7
剂型	jì-xíng	dosage form	15.1
济	jì	assist	4.5
寄生虫	jì-shēng-chóng	parasite	7.1
记录	jì-lù	record	15.8
记录下	jì-lù-xià	record; write down	15.8
记诵	jì-sòng	learn by heart	11.5
记忆力	jì-yì-lì	memory	5.6
既	jì	since	1.8
既不 ... 又不 ...	jì-bù ... yòu-bù ...	neither ... nor ...	7.7
既 ... 又 ...	jì ... yòu ...	... as well as ...	9.7
继续	jì-xù	continue	12.7
纪律	jì-lǜ	discipline	14.1
家	jiā	expert; author	15.8
家	jiā	house; family	6.8
家畜	jiā-chù	livestock	6.8
家族	jiā-zú	family	10.8
加	jiā	add	9.8
加工	jiā-gōng	process	16.2
加减	jiā-jiǎn	increase or decrease; modify	9.8
加剧	jiā-jù	increase	12.6

加强	jiā-qiáng	strengthen	3.8
加热	jiā-rè	add heat; heat	15.4
加入	jiā-rù	add	6.1
加上	jiā-shàng	add	12.2
加速	jiā-sù	accelerate; speed up	5.3
加以	jiā-yǐ	amend by; add	8.1
加以	jiā-yǐ	(an expression defining the immediately preceding statement as an object of the following verb; often intranslatable)	1.3
颊	jiá	lateral cheek	10.2
甲	jiǎ	first (in an enumeration)	2.8
假使	jiǎ-shǐ	if; when	5.2
假象	jiǎ-xiàng	false phenomena	12.2
价值	jià-zhí	value	3.8
坚	jiān	hard; solid	7.5
坚强	jiān-qiáng	vigorous	10.1
坚实	jiān-shí	hard	11.7
间	jiān	between; amidst; in	1.2
煎	jiān	boil (fast with strong heat)	15.3
煎熬	jiān-áo	boil	7.3
兼	jiān	together with	6.4
兼顾	jiān-gù	take into regard simultaneously	7.3
兼施	jiān-shī	apply simultaneously	12.1
艰	jiān	difficult	11.5
蹇涩	jiǎn-sè	impeded	6.2
简	jiǎn	short (in the sense of uncomplicated)	13.1
简单	jiǎn-dān	simple	8.6
简明	jiǎn-míng	simple and clear	9.8
减	jiǎn	decrease	9.8
减低	jiǎn-dī	reduce	16.2

减轻	jiǎn-qīng	alleviate	12.6
减少	jiǎn-shǎo	lessen; decrease	13.4
减退	jiǎn-tuì	decrease	7.5
减小	jiǎn-xiǎo	decrease	14.5
间隔	jiàn-gé	interval	3.8
间接	jiàn-jiē	indirect	2.6
见	jiàn	appear	1.5
见解	jiàn-jiě	perspective	15.8
健	jiàn	strengthen	1.7
健康	jiàn-kāng	health	6.8
健脾	jiàn-pí	strengthen the spleen	2.7
健全	jiàn-quán	be in order; perfect	4.2
渐	jiàn	gradually	13.7
溅起	jiàn-qǐ	splash	11.6
建泽泻	jiàn-zé-xiè	(the drug) zexie from (the province of Fu)jian	16.1
姜汁	jiāng-zhī	ginger extract	16.2
姜汁制	jiāng-zhī-zhì	processing with ginger extract	16.3
将	jiāng	(particle identifying the following expression as an object of the verb following that expression)	2.5
将军	jiāng-jūn	general; troop leader	4.2
强	jiàng	stiff	3.5
酱菜	jiàng-cài	food prepared with soy sauce	10.4
降	jiàng	sink	1.7
绛	jiàng	crimson	1.5
交	jiāo	unite	13.4
交替	jiāo-tì	alternate	9.4
脚气	jiǎo-qì	beriberi	13.2
脚肿	jiǎo-zhǒng	swollen legs	6.5
较	jiào	relatively; comparatively	6.6

叫做	jiào-zuò	be called; call	1.7
接触	jiē-chù	encounter	2.6
接近	jiē-jìn	be close to (some-one/something)	14.3
接受	jiē-shòu	receive	4.6
皆	jiē	all	5.2
阶段	jiē-duàn	phase	4.6
结实	jiē-shí	firm; strong; stable	8.5
节	jié	joint	6.5
节制	jié-zhì	restrain	7.4
捷	jié	quick	15.1
洁	jié	clean	7.5
结	jié	knot; cloddy	6.6
结果	jié-guǒ	result	6.4
结合	jié-hé	link; connect	2.6
结论	jié-lùn	conclusion	8.1
结束	jié-shù	finish; be finished	12.1
结胸	jié-xiōng	accumulation (of qi) in the chest	11.7
解	jiě	open; loosen	1.8
解	jiě	solve; end	10.7
解表	jiě-biǎo	open the exterior	1.8
解除	jiě-chú	remove; eliminate	9.2
解毒	jiě-dú	detoxify	13.5
解肌	jiě-jī	resolve the muscles	13.1
解决	jiě-jué	resolve	12.5
解释	jiě-shì	explain	1.2
解索	jiě-suǒ	untying a rope (pulse condition)	11.6
芥子	jiè-zǐ	mustard seed	15.1
借	jiè	make use of; borrow	2.1
借...来说	jiè ... lái shuō	state in terms of ...	2.1
筋	jīn	sinew	1.3

筋病	jīn-bìng	sinew illness	10.5
金	jīn	metal	2.1
金匮要略	jīn-guì-yào-lüè	(book title:) "Important (Pre-scriptions) from the Golden Chest"	14.4
金刃伤	jīn-rèn-shāng	injury from metal blades	7.7
今	jīn	now; today	14.4
津	jīn	jin humor	5.7
津液	jīn-yè	body liquids	5.7
紧	jǐn	tight	6.3
紧接	jǐn-jiē	follow next	13.1
仅	jǐn	only; merely	8.4
仅是 … 而已	jǐn-shì … ér-yǐ	be nothing but …	6.4
进	jìn	move into; eat	7.4
进入	jìn-rù	enter	8.3
进退	jìn-tuì	advance and retreat; come and go	11.5
进行	jìn-xíng	conduct; carry out	2.8
进一步	jìn-yī-bù	in a next step; then	4.6
近来	jìn-lái	recently	3.8
浸出液	jìn-chū-yè	maceration liquid	15.4
浸泡	jìn-pào	soak	16.3
浸取	jìn-qǔ	soak and extract	15.4
尽	jìn	completely	13.7
惊	jīng	fright	7.1
惊	jīng	tense	12.3
惊惕	jīng-tì	shock	4.2
精	jīng	essence; semen	1.4
精彩	jīng-cǎi	brilliant	10.1
精华	jīng-huá	essence	4.3
精力	jīng-lì	vigor	5.1
精力充沛	jīng-lì chōng-pèi	vigor	4.4

精气	jīng-qì	essential qi	1.3
精神	jīng-shén	spirit; mental	4.2
精神状态	jīng-shén-zhuàng-tài	mental state	10.8
精微	jīng-wēi	subtle	11.8
经	jīng	conduit	3.1
经	jīng	monthly period	4.2
经别	jīng-bié	conduit branches	3.1
经常	jīng-cháng	often	8.6
经典	jīng-diǎn	classic	14.4
经方	jīng-fāng	classic formulas	14.4
经过	jīng-guò	pass	6.8
经筋	jīng-jīn	conduit sinew	3.1
经络	jīng-luò	conduits and network (vessels)	3.1
经脉	jīng-mài	conduit vessels	3.1
经验	jīng-yàn	experience	15.8
静	jìng	rest; quietude	1.3
痉	jìng	spasm	10.5
胫酸	jìng-suān	pain in the lower leg	4.4
究竟	jiū-jìng	in the end; finally	8.7
纠正	jiū-zhèng	correct	16.4
久	jiǔ	long; chronic	8.5
灸	jiǔ	moxa	3.8
九窍	jiǔ-qiào	the nine orifices	3.3
酒	jiǔ	wine; liquor	15.1
酒剂	jiǔ-jì	alcoholic preparation	15.4
酒制	jiǔ-zhì	processing with alcohol	16.3
救	jiù	rescue	12.7
就	jiù	(particle indicating a subsequent process as an obvious consequence of a condition mentioned before)	1.2
就 ... 来说	jiù ... lái shuō	take ... as an example	2.5

就是	jiù-shì	that is	2.1
拘急	jū-jí	tension	12.2
居	jū	live	6.5
居住	jū-zhù	reside	7.6
橘子汁	jú-zǐ-zhī	orange juice	10.4
举	jǔ	lift	10.5
举例来说	jǔ-lì-lái shuō	to explain by way of example	2.7
拒	jù	resist; refuse	11.7
据	jù	evidence	10.4
具	jù	have	15.1
具备	jù-bèi	have	9.7
具体	jù-tǐ	concrete; specific	8.8
具有	jù-yǒu	possess; have	1.7
俱	jù	all	4.1
剧	jù	worsen	8.6
剧烈	jù-liè	violent	16.8
倦怠	juàn-dài	fatigue	6.4
觉	jué	perceive; feel	10.8
觉热	jué-rè	feeling of heat	9.4
决	jué	open; clear	4.7
决定	jué-dìng	decide	8.7
决断	jué-duàn	decide	4.5
绝	jué	break off	11.3
绝对	jué-duì	definitely	5.2
厥	jué	recede	9.4
厥冷	jué-lěng	recession (of yang qi giving rise to) cold	8.4
厥热交替	jué-rè-jiāo-tì	alternate occurrence of recession (of yang qi) and heat	9.4
厥阴	jué-yīn	ceasing yin	9.1
厥阴病	jué-yīn-bìng	ceasing yin illness	9.4
厥阴脉	jué-yīn-mài	ceasing yin vessel	9.4

均	jūn	all	2.4
均匀	jūn-yún	evenly	15.2
君	jūn	ruler	14.1
君火	jūn-huǒ	ruler fire	4.5
君药	jūn-yào	ruler drug	14.2
君主	jūn-zhǔ	lord	4.3
峻	jùn	drastic	12.7
峻补	jùn-bǔ	drastic supplementation	13.8
峻下	jùn-xià	drastic purgation	13.3

K

咯出	kǎ-chū	cough up	10.7
咯血	kǎ-xuè	haemoptysis	7.5
开	kāi	open	5.7
开始	kāi-shǐ	begin	10.7
开水	kāi-shuǐ	boiled water	15.1
看	kàn	view	7.6
看 ... 来 ...	kàn ... lái ...	observe ... to ...; (do something) on the basis of ...	14.2
看成	kàn-chéng	view as	12.1
看出	kàn-chū	recognize	2.1
抗争	kàng-zhēng	struggle	9.4
亢奋	kàng-fèn	agitated	9.1
亢旱	kàng-hàn	severe drought	6.8
亢进	kàng-jìn	hyperfunction	1.4
考虑	kǎo-lǜ	consider	5.8
靠	kào	depend on	5.4
柯韵伯	kē yùn-bó	(author's name) Ke Yunbo	9.8

科	kē	scientific or medical speciality	1.4
咳嗽	ké-sòu	cough	4.3
可	kě	can; be able	2.2
可会	kě-huì	definitely	11.5
可考	kě-kǎo	certainly	11.5
可以	kě-yǐ	can; be able	1.8
可知	kě-zhī	it can be realized	14.3
渴	kě	thirsty; thirst	5.8
渴饮	kě-yǐn	thirst	6.6
克	kè	restrain	2.1
克服	kè-fú	overcome	2.2
克制	kè-zhì	overcome	14.5
刻板	kè-bǎn	mechanical	15.6
客	kè	guest; take residence	12.3
客观	kè-guān	objective	1.1
课程	kè-chéng	branch of study; subject	3.1
肯定	kěn-dìng	confirm	14.4
空	kōng	empty	11.2
空洞	kōng-dòng	empty	5.6
恐	kǒng	fear	2.6
芤	kōu	(pulse condition resembling a) scallion stalk: hard outside, hollow inside	11.2
口	kǒu	mouth	2.6
口不作渴	kǒu-bù-zuò-kě	lack of thirst	8.4
口臭	kǒu-chòu	bad breath	6.7
口腹	kǒu-fù	eat; consume	7.4
口角	kǒu-jiǎo	corner of the mouth	10.5
口噤	kǒu-jìn	trismus	3.5
口噤不语	kǒu-jìn-bù-yǔ	clenched jaw and inability to speak	10.5
口渴	kǒu-kě	thirst	5.8

口苦	kǒu-kǔ	bitter feeling in the mouth	4.5
口内	kǒu-nèi	interior of the mouth	10.7
口气	kǒu-qì	breath	10.6
叩	kòu	knock against something	11.7
枯	kū	withered	10.4
哭泣	kū-qì	cry	7.1
苦	kǔ	bitter	1.7
苦味	kǔ-wèi	bitter flavor	16.6
块	kuài	piece	10.4
快	kuài	happy; comfortable	10.6
快	kuài	wellbeing	13.2
快慢	kuài-màn	fast and slow; speed	14.5
狂乱	kuáng-luàn	wild behavior	6.7
狂妄	kuáng-wàng	frantic	5.6
矿物	kuàng-wù	mineral	15.3
亏	kuī	loss	6.6
亏耗	kuī-hào	consumed; worn away; depleted; lost	5.1
亏损	kuī-sǔn	loss	14.7
困难	kùn-nán	difficulty	10.6

L

拉锯	lā-jù	bow saw	10.6
来	lái	come	2.4
来	lái	in order to	1.1
来往	lái-wǎng	come and go	11.3
懒言	lǎn-yán	laziness to talk	1.4
朗然	lǎng-rán	clear	9.8

劳	láo	fatigue	5.2
劳动	láo-dòng	work; toil	1.4
劳倦	láo-juàn	weariness from toil	8.3
劳热	láo-rè	exhaustion heat	13.4
牢	láo	tethered (pulse condition)	11.2
痨虫	láo-chóng	consumption worms	7.5
痨瘵	láo-zhài	consumption	7.5
老	lǎo	aged	10.4
乐	lè	joy	5.2
了	le	(particle defining the immediately preceding verb as past tense)	1.2
了	le	(resultative particle highlighting a new situation)	1.1
类	lèi	type; category	3.6
类似	lèi-sì	resemble	6.4
类推	lèi-tuī	deduce analogously	2.1
类型	lèi-xíng	type	1.4
泪	lèi	tears	5.8
冷	lěng	cold	1.4
冷浸	lěng-jìn	cold soaking	15.4
冷痛	lěng-tòng	cold pain	11.4
离	lí	leave; defy; go against	14.1
理	lǐ	principle; theory	15.6
理解	lǐ-jiě	understand	1.8
理论	lǐ-lùn	theory	1.1
理气	lǐ-qì	regulate the (flow of the) qi	2.7
理线	lǐ-xiàn	order threads	10.5
理由	lǐ-yóu	reason; cause	5.7
里	lǐ	inner	1.8
里寒	lǐ-hán	internal cold	11.4
里热	lǐ-rè	internal heat	13.5

里热（症）	lǐ-rè-(zhèng)	(pathocondition of) internal heat	13.5
里实	lǐ-shí	internal repletion	13.3
里实症	lǐ-shí-zhèng	pathoconditions of internal repletion	13.3
里症	lǐ-zhèng	pathoconditions affecting the body's interior	1.4
利	lì	benefit; advantage; (here:) maintain a free movement	3.1
利导	lì-dǎo	free (a passage) and guide (there)	13.7
利尿	lì-niào	free urination	13.7
利气	lì-qì	stimulate the qi (flow)	4.7
利湿	lì-shī	make liquid flow off	4.3
利水	lì-shuǐ	diuresis	13.7
利用	lì-yòng	use; make use of	14.3
例	lì	example	2.1
例如	lì-rú	for example	1.8
例证	lì-zhèng	example	14.4
痢疾	lì-ji	diarrhea	4.6
立	lì	stand	10.5
立方	lì-fāng	set up a formula	14.7
立即	lì-jí	immediate	7.2
粒	lì	(measure word for pellets)	15.1
力	lì	strength	14.5
力量	lì-liang	strength	4.3
联系	lián-xì	relationship	2.3
连	lián	tie; connect	11.6
连连	lián-lián	again and again; in rapid succession	11.6
凉	liáng	cool	1.6
凉法	liáng-fǎ	cooling (therapy) pattern	1.6
凉下	liáng-xià	cooling purging	8.8

362

凉性	liáng-xìng	cool nature	16.5
凉性药	liáng-xìng-yào	drug of cool nature	16.5
凉药	liáng-yào	cooling drugs	12.2
良	liáng	good	5.3
良久	liáng-jiǔ	long time	11.6
两	liǎng	two	1.2
两	liǎng	(weight; equal to 50 grams)	15.1
量	liàng	amount; dosage	14.8
疗法	liáo-fǎ	therapeutic method	4.6
疗效	liáo-xiào	therapeutic efficacy	14.4
燎原	liáo-yuán	prairie fire	6.7
了解	liǎo-jiě	understand; find out	10.8
列	liè	list; enumerate	4.1
列入	liè-rù	assign	9.1
列于	liè-yú	assign	9.1
裂纹	liè-wén	crackles	10.4
烈	liè	violent	16.8
烈日	liè-rì	burning sun	6.4
临床	lín-chuáng	clinical	1.1
临时	lín-shí	temporarily	10.1
临症	lín-zhèng	clinical (experience)	1.8
临症指南	lín-zhèng-zhǐ-nán	(book title) "Clinical Guideline"	15.8
淋浊	lín-zhuó	strangury and turbid (urine)	6.7
羚羊角	líng-yáng-jiǎo	antelope's horn	15.2
灵活	líng-huó	adaptable; flexible	1.1
另外	lìng-wài	in addition	15.3
另一	lìng-yī	another	5.1
另有	lìng-yǒu	in addition there is/are	5.1
留	liú	remain	3.5
留存	liú-cún	stay	12.4
流	liú	flow	15.4

流弊	liú-bì	unwanted effects; drawback	5.8
流窜	liú-cuàn	flow through ...	7.3
流利	liú-lì	flow	11.5
流入	liú-rù	flow into	6.5
流涕	liú-tì	flow of snivel	6.2
流通	liú-tōng	circulate; circulation	15.4
流行	liú-xíng	flow	3.3
六	liù	six	1.3
六百	liù-bǎi	six hundred	15.1
六变	liù-biàn	the six changes	8.1
六腑	liù-fǔ	the six palaces (i.e., gallbladder, bladder, stomach, small intestine, large intestine, triple burner)	1.3
六经	liù-jīng	the six conduits	9.1
六气	liù-qì	the six qi	6.1
六淫	liù-yín	the six excesses	6.1
龙胆草	lóng-dǎn-cǎo	(drug name) Gentiana scabra Bge.	1.7
聋	lóng	dumb	10.8
露	lù	dew	6.5
录	lù	record	11.5
陆续	lù-xù	successive	15.2
陆续配研	lù-xù-pèi-yán	successively additive grinding	15.2
偻	lǚ	bent	10.5
绿豆	lǜ-dòu	green bean	15.1
乱	luàn	wild	6.7
论	lùn	determine; discuss	3.4
论定	lùn-dìng	definitive statement	10.2
论断	lùn-duàn	evaluation	15.8
瘰疬	luǒ-lì	scrofula	7.3
络	luò	network (vessel); enclose	3.1

M

麻黄	má-huáng	(drug name) Ephedra sinica Staph.	3.7
麻黄汤	má-huáng-tāng	decoction with mahuang	14.2
麻木	má-mù	insensitivity	3.5
麻杏石甘汤	má-xìng-shí-gān-tāng	decoction with ma(huang), xing(ren), shi(gao) and gan(cao)	14.8
骂詈	mà-lì	curse	10.6
麦冬	mài-dōng	(drug name) Ophiopogon japonicus Ker-Gawl.	5.8
脉	mài	vessel	2.6
脉案	mài-àn	diagnostic record	15.6
脉来歇止	mài-lái-xiē-zhǐ	breaks in the arrival of the pulse	5.4
脉象	mài-xiàng	pulse quality	6.3
脉诊	mài-zhěn	pulse diagnosis	1.5
满	mǎn	fullness; full	7.5
满症	mǎn-zhèng	fullness pathocondition	11.7
慢慢	màn-màn	slow	11.5
慢性	màn-xìng	chronic	12.8
慢性病	màn-xìng-bìng	chronic illness	12.8
漫无	màn-wú	there is/are absolutely no ...	14.1
毛	máo	hair	1.3
毛发	máo-fà	hair; body hair	5.7
矛盾	máo-dùn	contradiction	12.5
枚	méi	(measure word for flat objects)	4.4
煤熏	méi-xūn	soot	10.5
没有	méi-yǒu	does not exist; there is no ...	3.8
没有意思的	méi-yǒu-yì-si-de	meaningless	8.7
眉棱骨	méi-léng-gǔ	superciliary ridge	3.7

眉目	méi-mù	brows and eyes; headers and titles; logical sequence of thoughts	9.8
莓苔	méi-tāi	moss coating	10.3
每一	měi-yī	each; any	1.3
每一个	měi-yī-gè	each	8.1
门	mén	(numerial for disciplines in science and medicine)	3.1
门类	mén-lèi	category	14.8
猛烈	měng-liè	violent	13.3
猛兽	měng-shòu	wild animal	7.7
梦	mèng	dream	6.7
梦遗	mèng-yí	dream emission	6.7
弥漫	mí-màn	penetrate; fill	9.2
米	mǐ	rice	7.5
米泔制	mǐ-gān-zhì	processing with water used for washing rice	16.3
米糊	mǐ-hú	rice paste	15.1
蜜	mì	honey	15.1
蜜蜂	mì-fēng	bee	15.8
密封	mì-fēng	thoroughly close	15.4
密切	mì-qiè	close	2.3
绵	mián	silk floss	11.2
面	miàn	face	6.5
面部	miàn-bù	face	7.5
面糊	miàn-hú	flour paste	15.1
面色	miàn-sè	facial color; complexion	7.5
敏感性	mǐn-gǎn-xìng	susceptibility; sensitivity	7.2
明	míng	clear	11.5
明白	míng-bái	understand	1.8
明朗	míng-lǎng	clear	10.1
明确	míng-què	make clear; emphasize	1.8

名	míng	name	5.1
名称	míng-chēng	designation; name	5.1
名词	míng-cí	designation; name; term	1.2
名字	míng-zì	name; designation	16.1
命门	mìng-mén	gate of life	4.4
摸床	mō-chuáng	touch gently the bedding	10.5
磨	mó	grind	13.7
末	mò	end	3.2
末期	mò-qī	final stage	9.4
没药	mò-yào	myrrha	15.2
谋虑	móu-lǜ	plotting and planning	4.2
某些	mǒu-xiē	certain (people, things, etc.)	13.2
某一	mǒu-yī	a specific	2.6
某种	mǒu-zhǒng	certain	2.4
母	mǔ	mother	2.1
木	mù	wood	2.1
目	mù	eye	2.6
目标	mù-biāo	objective	14.4
目赤	mù-chì	red eyes	6.7
目的	mù-dì	goal	8.7
目光	mù-guāng	eyesight	10.1
目前	mù-qián	today; at present	16.1
目无所见	mù-wú-suǒ-jiàn	impaired vision	4.4
目眩	mù-xuàn	dizziness	9.3

N

哪些	nǎ-xiē	which	15.7
哪一	nǎ-yī	which	3.6

纳	nà	take in	10.6
乃	nǎi	hence (often untranslatable)	11.2
乃是	nǎi-shì	that is; then it is ...	1.5
耐	nài	endure	1.4
南	nán	south	2.5
男子	nán-zǐ	male	4.4
难	nán	difficult	6.5
囊	náng	bag	11.7
桡骨	náo-gǔ	radius	11.1
蛲虫	náo-chóng	pinworm	7.5
脑	nǎo	brain	4.8
脑转	nǎo-zhuàn	spinning head; dizziness	4.4
恼怒	nǎo-nù	anger	4.2
呢	ne	(particle indicating a question that comes in the natural progression of discourse: "so, ..."?) here: which?	8.7
内	nèi	inner; inside; interior	1.3
内部	nèi-bù	inner section	1.3
内侧	nèi-cè	inner side	1.3
内经	nèi-jīng	(book title; abbreviation of:) [Huangdi Neijing] "Huang Di's Inner Classic"	9.1
内科	nèi-kē	internal medicine	3.8
内热	nèi-rè	inner heat	10.5
内热症	nèi-rè-zhèng	pathoconditions of inner heat	9.4
内容	nèi-róng	content	8.8
内伤	nèi-shāng	internal harm	6.6
内湿	nèi-shī	internal dampness	6.5
内实	nèi-shí	internal repletion	14.7
内庭	nèi-tíng	nei-ting (hole)	3.8
内消法	nèi-xiāo-fǎ	(therapeutic) pattern of internal elimination	1.8

368

内因	nèi-yīn	internal causes	6.1
内在	nèi-zài	internal	7.2
内脏	nèi-zàng	inner depots	2.8
内阻	nèi-zǔ	internal blockage	13.7
嫩	nèn	tender	10.4
能	néng	be able; can	1.3
能力	néng-lì	ability	1.3
腻	nì	slimy	5.8
逆	nì	countermovement; (in medical texts often used as an abbreviation for "qi flowing contrary to its normal direction")	14.6
年	nián	year	6.1
粘	nián	sticky	5.8
粘合物	nián-hé-wù	binder	15.1
粘腻	nián-nì	sticky	5.8
酿	niàng	produce	15.8
酿成	niàng-chéng	develop	7.5
尿	niào	urine	5.7
尿血	niào-xuè	bloody urine	5.7
凝结	níng-jié	coagulate	13.7
凝聚	níng-jù	congeal	5.8
凝滞	níng-zhì	congeal and stagnate	5.4
牛奶	niú-nǎi	cow's milk	10.4
脓	nóng	pus	1.8
浓缩	nóng-suō	thicken by boiling; concentrate	15.3
弄	nòng	make; do	7.8
怒	nù	anger	2.6
女劳疸	nǚ-láo-dǎn	exhaustion resulting from sexual intemperance	10.2
女子	nǚ-zǐ	female; woman	4.2
女子胞	nǚ-zǐ-bāo	womb; uterus	4.8

| 衄 | nǜ | spontaneous external bleeding | 5.7 |

O

呕	ǒu	vomit; retch	5.7
呕出	ǒu-chū	vomit	9.4
呕吐	ǒu-tù	vomiting	4.5
偶	ǒu	paired; even	14.6
偶方	ǒu-fāng	paired formula	14.5

P

怕	pà	fear	1.4
怕冷	pà-lěng	aversion to cold	1.4
排	pái	line	15.7
排	pái	emit	13.7
排除	pái-chú	eliminate	5.3
排空	pái-kōng	evacuation	3.8
排泄	pái-xiè	excrete	4.6
派	pài	group; (measure word)	9.2
旁	páng	side	10.3
膀胱	páng-guāng	urinary bladder	4.1
炮制	páo-zhì	process by roasting (general designation of the pharmaceutical processing of Chinese drugs)	16.2
泡	pào	steep	15.4

培土	péi-tǔ	heap soil	2.8
配成	pèi-chéng	combine	14.1
配合	pèi-hé	combination; matching	3.2
配合	pèi-hé	combine	16.8
配伍	pèi-wǔ	compose	14.1
配研	pèi-yán	grind while adding (individual substances)	15.2
膨	péng	inflation	7.5
脾	pí	spleen	2.6
脾病	pí-bìng	spleen illness	2.7
脾热病	pí-rè-bìng	spleen heat illness	10.2
脾泻	pí-xiè	spleen drainage	2.8
脾虚	pí-xū	spleen depletion	7.4
脾阳	pí-yáng	the spleen-yang	5.8
疲	pí	tired	10.1
疲乏	pí-fá	fatigue	4.3
疲倦	pí-juàn	fatigue	1.4
疲劳	pí-láo	fatigue	5.4
皮	pí	skin	1.3
皮肤	pí-fū	skin	6.5
痞	pǐ	block	14.7
痞闷	pǐ-mèn	blocks and chest pressure	5.3
痞气	pǐ-qì	blocked qi	11.7
譬如	pì-rú	for example	7.7
偏	piān	one-sided	5.4
偏亢	piān-kàng	unilaterally excessive	4.5
偏凉	piān-liáng	unilaterally cool (qi)	16.5
偏胜	piān-shèng	unilateral dominance	14.7
偏盛	piān-shèng	unilateral flourishing	16.4
偏衰	piān-shuāi	unilaterial weakness	16.4
偏温	piān-wēn	unilaterally warm (qi)	16.5
贫	pín	poor; lacking	1.4

贫血	pín-xuè	anemia	1.4
平	pīng	pacify	12.3
平	píng	even; level; calm	1.8
平补	píng-bǔ	balanced supplementation	13.8
平喘	píng-chuǎn	calm panting	12.5
平肝	píng-gān	calm the liver	1.8
平衡	píng-héng	balance	2.3
平静	píng-jìng	quiet	10.1
平气	píng-qì	balanced qi	16.5
平日	píng-rì	daily	15.8
平胃散	píng-wèi-sǎn	powder calming down the stomach	14.7
凭	píng	by means of	10.1
破伤风	pò-shāng-fēng	tetanus	7.7
迫	pò	agitated	6.7
普遍	pǔ-biàn	universal; ubiquitous; general	1.2
普通	pǔ-tōng	general	6.8

Q

期	qī	phase	9.2
七	qī	seven	10.8
七方	qī-fāng	the seven formulas	14.5
七怪脉	qī-guài-mài	the seven uncommon pulses	11.6
七窍	qī-qiào	the seven orifices	2.6
七情	qī-qíng	seven affects	7.1
七情病	qī-qíng-bìng	illnesses (caused) by the seven affects	7.2
其	qí	his; her; its	2.8

其次	qí-cì	furthermore; next	10.3
其实	qí-shí	in fact	7.6
其它	qí-tā	others	2.1
其他	qí-tā	others	7.6
其余	qí-yú	the remaining	6.1
其中	qí-zhōng	among them	3.2
奇	qí	extraordinarily	10.7
奇恒	qí-héng	extraordinary	4.8
奇经八脉	qí-jīng-bā-mài	the eight extraordinary conduit vessels	3.1
齐	qí	regular	11.3
起	qǐ	bring forth; set off	1.8
起来	qǐ-lái	raise; mention	4.1
起来	qǐ-lái	(particle emphasizing a moving towards above or an initial movement indicated by the immediately preceding verb)	2.5
起有	qǐ-yǒu	fulfill	3.1
启发	qǐ-fā	enlighten	15.8
器官	qì-guān	organ	8.2
气	qì	qi	1.3
气	qì	qi (drug quality)	1.7
气	qì	breath	1.4
气喘	qì-chuǎn	panting	4.3
气促	qì-cù	panting	7.5
气短	qì-duǎn	shortness of breath	8.5
气分	qì-fèn	qi section	5.3
气分热	qì-fèn-rè	heat in the qi section	13.5
气膈	qì-gé	qi blockage	5.3
气臌	qì-gǔ	qi bloating	5.3
气候	qì-hòu	climate	2.5
气化	qì-huà	qi transformation	4.7

气机	qì-jī	qi movement	5.3
气淋	qì-lín	qi strangury	5.3
气色	qì-sè	complexion	10.1
气体	qì-tǐ	gas	5.3
气味	qì-wèi	smell	10.6
气虚	qì-xū	qi depletion	10.2
气壅	qì-yōng	qi obstruction	5.3
气郁	qì-yù	qi stagnation	5.3
气胀	qì-zhàng	distension resulting from gas	11.7
气滞	qì-zhì	qi sluggishness	5.3
牵制	qiān-zhì	restrain	16.8
千	qiān	thousand	15.1
钱	qián	(weight; equal to 5 grams)	15.1
前	qián	first; former	1.2
前	qián	before	2.7
前额	qián-é	forehead	3.7
前人	qián-rén	people of former times	1.2
潜伏	qián-fú	hidden; invisible	1.4
浅	qiǎn	shallow; superficial	3.5
浅部	qiǎn-bù	surface region	3.2
强	qiáng	strong; strength	4.4
强烈	qiáng-liè	strong	15.2
强盛	qiáng-shèng	strength and abundance	8.5
强壮	qiáng-zhuàng	strengthen; be strong	13.8
憔悴	qiáo-cuì	wither	5.7
且	qiě	even	6.3
切	qiè	palpate	10.1
切	qiè	very; certainly	11.8
切忌	qiè-jì	definitely not do/be something	11.8
切脉	qiè-mài	feel the pulse	11.1
切宜	qiè-yí	it is necessary	11.8

切诊	qiè-zhěn	palpation	11.1
侵	qīn	intrude	9.2
侵犯	qīn-fàn	intrude	4.2
侵害	qīn-hài	enter and cause harm	7.6
侵入	qīn-rù	invade	7.7
亲	qīn	relatives	10.6
亲自	qīn-zì	personal	16.6
琴弦	qín-xián	lute string	11.3
青	qīng	virid	1.5
青果	qīng-guǒ	olives	10.4
轻	qīng	light; minor	3.5
轻按	qīng-àn	press lightly	11.1
轻减	qīng-jiǎn	lessen	12.6
轻浅	qīng-qiǎn	mild; light	5.8
轻微	qīng-wēi	mild; light	6.2
轻扬	qīng-yáng	lift	13.1
倾	qīng	tip up; overturn; pour out	13.2
倾出	qīng-chū	pour off	15.5
倾向	qīng-xiàng	tendency	1.4
清	qīng	clear	4.3
清	qīng	cool	1.8
清补	qīng-bǔ	cool supplementation	13.8
清楚	qīng-chu	clear	7.8
清代	qīng-dài	the Qing dynasty (1644-1912)	14.4
清法	qīng-fǎ	the pattern of cooling	13.5
清谷	qīng-gǔ	undigested food	9.4
清化	qīng-huà	transformation by means of cooling	13.7
清降法	qīng-jiàng-fǎ	(therapeutic) pattern for cooling and subduing (heat)	1.8
清解	qīng-jiě	cooling through opening	1.8

清解法	qīng-jiě-fǎ	pattern of resolution through cooling	13.5
清解药	qīng-jiě-yào	cooling drugs	12.6
清净	qīng-jìng	purity	4.5
清凉	qīng-liáng	cool	13.1
清凉剂	qīng-liáng-jì	cooling prescription	7.8
清热	qīng-rè	cool the heat	1.8
清热药	qīng-rè-yào	drugs cooling heat	16.7
清水	qīng-shuǐ	clear water	6.3
情怀	qíng-huái	emotion	10.6
情况	qíng-kuàng	condition	1.8
情志	qíng-zhì	emotional	4.2
情志病	qíng-zhì-bìng	emotional illness	7.1
秋	qiū	autumn	2.5
秋季	qiū-jì	autumn	6.6
秋天	qiū-tiān	autumn	6.8
秋燥	qiū-zào	autumn dryness	6.6
求	qiú	search	12.4
求得	qiú-de	find out	7.8
趋势	qū-shì	tend; tendency	13.3
区别	qū-bié	distinguish	1.4
区域	qū-yù	region	9.1
躯干	qū-gàn	trunk	3.3
屈	qū	bend	5.7
驱	qū	chase away	13.4
驱除	qū-chú	eliminate	12.1
祛	qū	dispell	6.3
祛除	qū-chú	eliminate	13.6
祛寒药	qū-hán-yào	drugs eliminating cold	16.7
祛邪	qū-xié	eliminate the evil	12.5
取	qǔ	get (something as a result of an investigation); notice	11.2

取	qǔ	use	15.1
取	qǔ	take	12.3
去	qù	go; in order to	1.2
去	qù	remove	15.4
去掉	qù-diào	eliminate	12.4
去膜	qù-mó	remove the skin	10.4
颧	quán	cheek	7.5
权宜之计	quán-yí-zhī-jì	expediency	12.7
泉源	quán-yuán	source	7.4
全	quán	total	16.1
全部	quán-bù	entirety	8.1
全面	quán-miàn	complete; total; entirety	9.8
全身	quán-shēn	the entire body	3.1
痊愈	quán-yù	cure; heal	9.5
蜷曲	quán-qū	bent	10.5
缺少	quē-shǎo	deficiency	5.8
却	què	retreat; leave	12.5
确定	què-dìng	decision; decide	8.8
雀啄	què-zhuó	pecking bird (pulse condition)	11.6
群	qún	group	8.7

R

然	rán	like; as if	11.2
然而	rán-ér	still; however	16.4
然后	rán-hòu	then; afterwards	11.8
染	rǎn	infect	6.8
染舌	rǎn-shé	stained tongue	10.4

攘	rǎng	defense; defend	13.4
热	rè	hot; heat	1.4
热病	rè-bìng	illnesses caused by heat	6.4
热度	rè-dù	degree of fever	12.6
热结	rè-jié	heat accumulations	13.3
热浸	rè-jìn	hot soaking	15.4
热利	rè-lì	heat type diarrhea	9.4
热盛	rè-shèng	extreme heat	10.6
热痰	rè-tán	heat-phlegm	7.3
热象	rè-xiàng	heat signs	1.6
热邪	rè-xié	heat evil	5.4
热性	rè-xìng	hot nature	1.4
热性病	rè-xìng-bìng	heat type illness	5.8
热性药	rè-xìng-yào	drug of hot nature	16.4
热药	rè-yào	hot drugs	12.2
热阵	rè-zhèn	heating array	14.7
热症	rè-zhèng	pathoconditions of heat	1.4
人	rén	man	1.2
人身	rén-shēn	human body	4.5
人体组织	rén-tǐ-zǔ-zhī	the human organism	2.5
人体	rén-tǐ	the human body	1.3
忍	rěn	bear; endure	13.2
任何	rèn-hé	each; any	7.8
任何一 ... 都	rèn-hé yī ... dōu	everybody; each	2.1
认识	rèn-shi	recognize; cognition	5.1
认识到	rèn-shi-dào	realize; recognize	16.6
认为	rèn-wéi	deem; think; consider; hold	1.3
仍	réng	still	8.3
仍旧	réng-jiù	as before; unchanged	16.3
仍然	réng-rán	nevertheless; still	12.2
日	rì	sun	1.2

日渐	rì-jiàn	daily; day by day	6.3
荣	róng	flourishing	10.4
熔合	róng-hé	melt	15.3
溶剂	róng-jì	solvent	15.4
容易	róng-yì	simple	7.6
柔肝	róu-gān	emolliate the liver	2.7
肉	ròu	flesh	1.3
肉桂	ròu-guì	(drug name) Cinnamomum cassia Presl.	1.7
蠕动	rú-dòng	peristalsis	3.8
如	rú	for example; e.g.; be like	1.2
如 ... 便是	rú ... biàn-shì	as for example	14.5
如果	rú-guǒ	if; when	6.1
如何 (来)	rú-hé (lái)	how to	8.8
如环无端	rú huán wú duān	like a ring without end	3.3
如前所说	rú-qián-suǒ-shuō	as stated before	16.7
如同	rú-tóng	equal to; as if	12.7
濡	rú	moisten	3.1
濡	rú	soft (pulse condition)	11.2
乳钵	rǔ-bō	mortar	15.2
乳香	rǔ-xiāng	olibanum	15.2
乳汁制	rǔ-zhī-zhì	processing with milk	16.3
入	rù	enter	3.3
润	rùn	moist; moisten	6.6
润泽	rùn-zé	moisten	4.6
若	ruò	if; when	7.3
弱	ruò	weak	2.3

S

塞	sāi	obstruction	12.3
三	sān	three	3.7
三拗汤	sān-ǎo-tāng	decoction with the three untreated (ingredients)	14.8
三部	sān-bù	the three sections (at the wrists where the pulse can be felt)	11.1
三焦	sān-jiāo	triple burner	4.1
三阳	sān-yáng	the three yang (conduits)	9.1
三阳病	sān-yáng-bìng	illnesses of the three yang (conduits)	9.3
三阴	sān-yīn	the three yin (conduits)	9.1
三阴病	sān-yīn-bìng	illnesses of the three yin (conduits)	9.3
三阴交	sān-yīn-jiāo	san-yin-jiao (hole)	3.8
三因	sān-yīn	the three causes (of illness)	7.7
散	sǎn	powder	15.1
散剂	sǎn-jì	powder preparation	15.2
散乱	sǎn-luàn	disturbed	10.5
散	sàn	disperse	1.7
散阵	sàn-zhèn	dispersing array	14.7
色	sè	color	1.5
色欲	sè-yù	sexual desire	7.7
涩	sè	rough	1.5
砂仁	shā-rén	(drug name) Amomum xanthioides Wall.	1.7
煽张	shān-zhāng	be widened in excitement	10.5
善	shàn	tend to	6.2
善忘	shàn-wàng	forgetfulness	4.2
善于	shàn-yú	be good for; be well-suited for	16.7
伤	shāng	harm	1.8

380

伤风	shāng-fēng	harm caused by wind	1.8
伤害	shāng-hài	harm; damage	7.7
伤寒	shāng-hán	harm caused by cold	6.3
伤寒贯珠集	shāng-hán-guàn-zhū-jí	(book title:) "Threaded Pearls on Harm caused by Cold"	9.8
伤寒来苏集	shāng-hán-lái-sū-jí	(book title:) "Comprehensive Collection on Harm caused by Cold"	9.8
伤寒论	shāng-hán-lùn	(book title) "On Harm Caused by Cold"	9.1
伤食	shāng-shí	harm (caused by) food	7.4
伤暑	shāng-shǔ	harm from summerheat	11.4
商	shāng	consider	12.7
上	shàng	on; in	1.3
上党	shàng-dǎng	(place name) Shangdang	16.1
上的	shàng-de	being present in ...; concerning	1.1
上焦	shàng-jiāo	the upper burner	1.3
上面	shàng-miàn	above	14.4
上逆	shàng-nì	rise	4.2
上扰	shàng-rǎo	rise to cause harassment above	13.5
上升	shàng-shēng	rise	5.8
上述	shàng-shù	mentioned above	2.3
上所述	shàng-suǒ-shù	said above	4.8
上涌	shàng-yǒng	gush upwards	13.2
尚	shàng	still	3.7
稍	shāo	few; little	3.5
少	shǎo	few; little	1.4
少气	shǎo-qì	short of breath	1.4
少许	shǎo-xǔ	a little; small amount	12.2
少阳	shào-yáng	minor yang	9.1
少阳经	shào-yáng-jīng	minor yang conduit	3.7
少阳脉	shào-yáng-mài	minor yang vessel	9.3

少阴	shào-yīn	minor yin	9.1
少阴病	shào-yīn-bìng	minor yin illness	9.4
少阴脉	shào-yīn-mài	minor yin vessel	9.4
舌	shé	tongue	1.5
舌根	shé-gēn	base of the tongue	10.3
舌光	shé-guāng	tongue gloss	10.4
舌尖	shé-jiān	tip of the tongue	10.3
舌强	shé-jiàng	stiffness of the tongue	3.5
舌苔	shé-tāi	tongue coating	1.5
舌诊	shé-zhěn	tongue diagnosis	1.5
舌质	shé-zhì	tongue substance	1.5
麝香	shè-xiāng	musk	15.2
伸	shēn	stretch	5.7
身	shēn	body	2.4
身热	shēn-rè	body heat	6.4
身疼	shēn-téng	body pains	8.2
身体	shēn-tǐ	body	5.7
深	shēn	deep	3.5
深部	shēn-bù	deep-lying regions	3.2
神	shén	spirit	3.5
神病	shén-bìng	spirit illness	5.6
神昏	shén-hūn	mental confusion	6.7
神见	shén-jiàn	perfect understanding	10.8
神疲	shén-pí	mental weakness	8.5
神气	shén-qì	spirit qi	10.5
神思	shén-sī	mental state	10.1
神识	shén-zhì	mental	4.2
神志	shén-zhì	mind	7.1
神志昏糊	shén-zhì-hūn-hú	mental confusion	9.2
甚	shèn	severe	7.5
甚至	shèn-zhì	even; possibly going as far as to	4.2

肾	shèn	kidneys	1.7
肾亏	shèn-kuī	kidney deficiency	5.5
肾气	shèn-qì	kidney qi	4.7
肾热病	shèn-rè-bìng	kidney heat illness	10.2
肾虚	shèn-xū	kidney depletion	4.4
肾脏	shèn-zàng	kidneys	4.4
慎	shèn	careful	13.5
渗	shèn	seep	15.3
声	shēng	sound	10.6
声音	shēng-yīn	voice	8.5
生	shēng	create; engender	2.1
生	shēng	raw	16.2
生出	shēng-chū	generate	7.8
生化	shēng-huà	lifecycle	2.5
生活	shēng-huó	life	7.2
生机	shēng-jī	life processes	11.6
生金	shēng-jīn	generate metal	2.8
生津药	shēng-jīn-yào	drugs generating humor	5.8
生津液	shēng-jīn-yè	generate body liquids	13.8
生理	shēng-lǐ	physiology	1.1
生命	shēng-mìng	life; vital	4.2
生气	shēng-qì	vital qi	11.7
生药	shēng-yào	raw drug	16.2
生长	shēng-zhǎng	growth	5.5
生殖	shēng-zhí	reproduction	4.2
升	shēng	ascend	1.7
升华	shēng-huá	sublimate	15.3
升提	shēng-tí	rise	16.3
盛	shèng	abundant	2.3
盛衰	shèng-shuāi	flourishing and frailty	8.5
胜	shèng	dominate	1.6

胜任	shèng-rèn	stand (something)	14.5
师	shī	teacher	15.8
失	shī	miss	14.5
失常	shī-cháng	irregular	4.2
失眠	shī-mián	insomnia	4.2
失却	shī-què	miss entirely	14.5
失调	shī-tiáo	lose rhythm	5.4
失血	shī-xuè	loss of blood	7.8
失音	shī-yīn	loss of voice	7.5
湿	shī	dampness	2.5
湿气	shī-qì	dampness qi	6.4
湿热	shī-rè	dampness and heat	7.5
湿痰	shī-tán	dampness-phlegm	7.3
湿邪	shī-xié	dampness evil	6.1
十	shí	ten	10.8
十二	shí-èr	twelve	3.1
十分	shí-fēn	maximum	12.1
十问	shí-wèn	the ten (diagnostic) questions	10.8
十问歌	shí-wèn-gē	the Poem of the Ten (diagnostic) Questions	10.8
石膏	shí-gāo	(drug name) gypsum	14.8
石斛	shí-hú	(drug name) Dendrobium nobile Lindl.	5.8
时	shí	while; during	5.3
时	shí	time	2.4
时	shí	from time to time	10.6
时病	shí-bìng	seasonal illness	10.7
时方	shí-fāng	formulas (introduced in later) times	14.4
时候	shí-hòu	time	5.6
时间	shí-jiān	time	3.8
时期	shí-qī	period of time	6.8

时气	shí-qì	seasonal qi	6.6
时邪	shí-xié	seasonal evil	10.3
时症	shí-zhèng	seasonal pathocondition	12.8
食	shí	food; meal	4.3
食积	shí-jī	food accumulation	7.5
食品	shí-pǐn	food items	6.5
食物	shí-wù	food	4.3
食物中毒	shí-wù-zhòng-dú	food poisoning	7.7
食欲	shí-yù	appetite	7.5
食指	shí-zhǐ	index finger	11.1
食滞	shí-zhì	food blockage	10.7
实	shí	replete (pulse condition)	11.2
实	shí	fact; reality	1.8
实	shí	repletion	1.8
实火	shí-huǒ	repletion fire	6.7
实际	shí-jì	reality	1.1
实际上	shí-jì-shàng	in reality	8.1
实践	shí-jiàn	practice	1.1
实热	shí-rè	repletion heat	10.2
实热症	shí-rè-zhèng	pathoconditions of repletion heat	13.3
实邪	shí-xié	solid evil	13.2
实验	shí-yàn	experiment; experimental	3.8
实有	shí-yǒu	fact	1.8
实症	shí-zhèng	pathocondition of repletion	8.5
实质上	shí-zhì-shàng	in essence; in reality	12.2
识	shí	recognize	5.6
史	shǐ	history	10.8
矢气	shǐ-qì	flatulence	10.7
使	shǐ	cause	2.3
使	shǐ	if; given	14.1
使	shǐ	messenger	14.1

使药	shǐ-yào	messenger drug	14.3
使用	shǐ-yòng	apply	12.1
始	shǐ	begin	11.2
事	shì	affair	11.5
事物	shì-wù	thing; item	1.2
势	shì	force	6.7
势必	shì-bì	inevitable	12.4
是	shì	be; is	1.2
是	shì	(particle emphasizing the state-ment of the following verb)	3.2
是	shì	this	7.8
是否	shì-fǒu ...	whether; whether ... or not	11.4
嗜	shì	take delight in	6.5
适	shì	suitable	15.3
适当	shì-dàng	appropriate	15.5
适应	shì-yìng	be suited for	14.8
适应范围	shì-yìng-fàn-wéi	scope of indications	16.7
适用	shì-yòng	suitable	16.2
视	shì	observe; behold	15.5
视...而定	shì ... ér dìng	determine on the basis of ...	15.7
视觉	shì-jué	visual sense	10.1
收	shōu	shrink	2.5
收敛法	shōu-liǎn-fǎ	contracting (therapy) pattern	12.2
收敛	shōu-liǎn	draw together; contract	16.3
收摄	shōu-shè	acquire	5.3
收缩	shōu-suō	contraction	3.8
收引	shōu-yǐn	draw together	6.3
手	shǒu	hand	3.6
手背	shǒu-bèi	back of the hand	11.7
手心	shǒu-xīn	palm	11.7
手续	shǒu-xù	procedure	15.2
手指	shǒu-zhǐ	finger	13.2

386

首乌	shǒu-wū	(drug name) Polygonum multiflorum Thunb.	1.7
首先	shǒu-xiān	first	7.8
受	shòu	receive	4.2
受到	shòu-dào	receive	4.2
受纳	shòu-nà	intake	4.5
瘦	shòu	emaciated	7.5
兽	shòu	quadrupeds; animals	7.7
输送	shū-sòng	transportation	4.6
舒	shū	free; open	2.7
舒畅	shū-chàng	be unimpeded	2.7
舒缓法	shū-huǎn-fǎ	relaxing (therapy) pattern	12.2
舒筋	shū-jīn	relax the sinews	15.4
疏	shū	distant	10.6
疏畅	shū-chàng	open; make passable	4.7
疏肝	shū-gān	clear the liver	2.7
疏解	shū-jiě	course and open	13.1
疏浚	shū-jùn	dredge	12.7
疏散	shū-sàn	disperse; dispersion	1.8
疏通	shū-tōng	dredge; make passable	4.7
书	shū	text	5.5
书写	shū-xiě	write down	15.7
熟	shú	processed	16.2
熟地	shú-dì	(drug name) Rehmannia glutinosa (Gaertn.) Libosch.	16.2
熟悉	shú-xī	be familiar with	3.6
暑	shǔ	summerheat	2.5
暑病	shǔ-bìng	illnesses caused by summerheat	6.4
暑热	shǔ-rè	summerheat-heat	6.4
暑湿	shǔ-shī	summerheat-dampness	6.4
暑邪	shǔ-xié	summerheat evil	6.1
属	shǔ	belong to	1.4

属性	shǔ-xìng	attribute	1.2
属于	shǔ-yú	be associated with; belong to	1.3
数	shù	number	1.5
数次	shù-cì	several times; repeatedly	9.3
衰	shuāi	weak	11.3
衰竭	shuāi-jié	weakness	11.6
衰弱	shuāi-ruò	weak	1.4
衰退	shuāi-tuì	weaken	4.4
帅	shuài	commander	5.2
双	shuāng	both	14.6
双数	shuāng-shù	even numbers	14.6
水	shuǐ	water	1.2
水道	shuǐ-dào	water way	4.7
水分	shuǐ-fèn	water (fluid) content	5.7
水谷	shuǐ-gǔ	water and grain; liquid and solid food	4.1
水浸	shuǐ-jìn	soak in water	15.3
水面	shuǐ-miàn	water surface	11.6
水气	shuǐ-qì	water qi	10.2
水湿	shuǐ-shī	liquid	4.3
水液	shuǐ-yè	liquid	4.6
水胀	shuǐ-zhàng	distension resulting from water	11.7
睡眠	shuì-mián	sleep	6.7
顺	shùn	appropriate	13.7
顺从	shùn-cóng	go along with	12.2
说成	shuō-chéng	designate as; speak of	16.5
说法	shuō-fǎ	opinion; statement	5.2
说明	shuō-míng	explain	1.1
数	shuò	frequent; accelerated	1.5
思	sī	thought	2.6
思卧	sī-wò	sleepiness	4.4
思想	sī-xiǎng	thought; idea	1.1

司	sī	regulate	4.3
丝	sī	silk	11.5
死	sǐ	die	6.8
死亡	sǐ-wáng	die	12.1
四	sì	four	1.4
四百	sì-bǎi	four hundred	15.1
四川	sì-chuān	(name of province) Sichuan	16.1
四季	sì-jì	the four seasons	6.1
四逆汤	sì-nì-tāng	decoction against countermovement (of qi in the) four (limbs)	14.6
四气	sì-qì	thc four qi	16.5
四项	sì-xiàng	the four components (in structuring a prescription)	14.1
四诊	sì-zhěn	the four examinations	10.1
四肢	sì-zhī	the four limbs	3.2
四周	sì-zhōu	in all four directions; all around	10.2
似	sì	appear like	4.8
俟	sì	wait; only then	12.7
松	sōng	dry; flaky	10.4
松弛	sōng-chí	slacken	8.5
溲	sōu	urinate; urine	6.7
溲少	sōu-shǎo	scant urine	6.5
苏醒	sū-xǐng	regain consciousness	6.2
俗	sú	commonly	7.5
俗称	sú-chēng	be commonly called	15.1
俗呼	sú-hū	be commonly called	15.4
索	sù	permanent	7.5
素	sù	since birth	13.5
速	sù	fast	11.6
粟粒	sù-lì	millet grain	7.5
宿粪	sù-fèn	faeces staying (in the intestines)	13.3

宿食	sù-shí	undigested food	10.7
肃	sù	lofty	4.3
肃	sù	free; unimpeded	7.3
酸	suān	sour	1.7
酸楚	suān-chǔ	ache	12.6
酸软	suān-ruǎn	painful and weak	8.2
酸味	suān-wèi	sour flavor	16.6
算	suàn	consider; consider as	12.1
虽	suī	even though	4.5
虽然	suī-rán	even though	10.1
随	suí	follow; afterwards; subsequently	12.4
随即	suí-jí	soon afterwards	11.6
髓	suǐ	marrow	4.8
损害	sǔn-hài	injury	7.7
损伤	sǔn-shāng	injury; injure	7.7
损失	sǔn-shī	lose	1.4
缩短	suō-duǎn	shorten	3.8
缩缩	suō-suō	shrunken	11.5
锁喉症	suǒ-hóu-zhèng	pathocondition of "obstructed throat"	13.2
所	suǒ	(relative pronoun)	1.2
所属	suǒ-shǔ	associated; belonging	3.5
所说的	suǒ-shuō-de	so-called	5.7
所谓	suǒ-wèi	so-called	3.3
所以	suǒ-yǐ	hence	1.8
... 所致	... suǒ-zhì	be caused by ...	4.3

T

他	tā	he/she; his/her	15.8
它	tā	it	1.1
它的	tā-de	its (possessive pronoun; genitive singular)	3.1
它们	tā-men	they	2.3
胎	tāi	fetus	4.8
苔	tāi	coating	10.3
太	tài	too much	14.3
太息	tài-xī	deep sigh	7.1
太阳	tài-yáng	major yang	9.1
太阳病	tài-yáng-bìng	major yang illness	9.2
太阳经	tài-yáng-jīng	major yang conduit	3.7
太阳脉	tài-yáng-mài	major yang vessel	9.2
太阴	tài-yīn	major yin	9.1
太阴病	tài-yīn-bìng	major yin illness	9.3
太阴脉	tài-yīn-mài	major yin vessel	9.3
贪	tān	gluttonous	7.4
坛	tán	jar	15.4
弹石	tán-shí	flicking a stone (pulse condition)	11.6
痰	tán	phlegm	6.5
痰喘	tán-chuǎn	phlegm panting	10.2
痰热	tán-rè	phlegm heat	13.7
痰饮	tán-yǐn	phlegm drink	5.8
痰浊	tán-zhuó	phlegm-turbidity	7.3
痰阻	tán-zǔ	phlegm obstruction	10.6
谈不到	tán-bù-dào	cannot be said; be impossible	4.5
探	tàn	investigate	12.5
探求	tàn-qiú	search; investigate	11.4

探吐	tàn-tù	vomiting (induced) by poking (into the throat)	13.2
叹息	tàn-xī	sigh	10.6
炭	tàn	coal	16.2
汤	tāng	hot liquid	8.4
汤火伤	tāng-huǒ-shāng	injury from hot liquid and fire	7.7
汤剂	tāng-jì	decoction preparation	15.5
汤水	tāng-shuǐ	hot water	7.7
溏薄	táng-bó	semiliquid	7.4
倘 ... 便	tǎng ... biàn	if ..., then	14.8
倘 ... 则	tǎng ... zé	if ..., then	4.3
烫伤	tàng-shāng	scalding	7.7
套	tào	(a totality of something that consists of individual parts)	15.6
特	tè	special	16.1
特别	tè-bié	particular; special	5.2
特长	tè-cháng	strength; advantage	9.8
特点	tè-diǎn	characteristic	4.4
特殊	tè-shū	specific; special	1.3
特有	tè-yǒu	characteristic; unique	1.3
特征	tè-zhēng	characteristic	9.4
疼痛	téng-tòng	pain	3.7
提出	tí-chū	propose	5.2
提纲挈领	tí-gāng-qiè-lǐng	concentrate on the essential	9.8
提高	tí-gāo	increase	16.1
体	tǐ	substance; body	3.3
体表	tǐ-biǎo	the body's exterior	1.3
体会	tǐ-huì	understand (by personal experience rather than rationally); understanding	5.2
体力	tǐ-lì	physical strength	5.5
体内	tǐ-nèi	the body's interior	1.3

体系	tǐ-xì	system	1.1
体质	tǐ-zhì	physical constitution	5.4
体重	tǐ-zhòng	heaviness of the body	6.4
体状	tǐ-zhuàng	physical appearance	1.5
涕	tì	snivel	5.8
天	tiān	heaven	1.2
天花粉	tiān-huā-fěn	(drug name) Trichosanthes kirilowii Maxim.	5.8
天雨	tiān-yǔ	rain	6.5
填骨髓	tián-gǔ-suí	fill the bone marrow	13.8
田野	tián-yě	open field	6.4
甜	tián	sweet	6.5
挑取	tiāo-qǔ	take	15.3
条畅	tiáo-chàng	pass through; be unimpeded	2.7
条件	tiáo-jiàn	condition; precondition	2.3
调	tiáo	regulate	4.2
调和	tiáo-he	regulate	13.4
调节	tiáo-jié	regulate	3.2
调理	tiáo-lǐ	regulate	13.4
调养	tiáo-yǎng	regulate nourishment	5.5
调整	tiáo-zhěng	regulate	16.4
迢迢	tiáo-tiáo	stretched; distant	11.5
贴	tiē	paste	15.3
听觉	tīng-jué	sense of hearing	10.6
听取	tīng-qǔ	listen	10.6
停	tíng	stagnate	13.7
停水	tíng-shuǐ	stagnant water	4.7
停滞	tíng-zhì	stagnate	4.3
通	tōng	penetrate; make passable	12.3
通导	tōng-dǎo	purge	4.6
通过	tōng-guò	pass through	1.8
通过	tōng-guò	by way of	16.6

通利	tōng-lì	open for passage	5.3
通路	tōng-lù	pathway; thoroughfare	3.3
同	tóng	identical; similar	2.5
同	tóng	common	5.7
同时	tóng-shí	at the same time	2.5
同样	tóng-yàng	likewise	2.7
同一	tóng-yī	identical	7.8
童便制	tóng-biàn-zhì	processing with boys' urine	16.3
统	tǒng	govern	4.3
统帅	tǒng-shuài	commander	5.1
统一	tǒng-yī	united; unity	1.2
痛	tòng	pain	3.5
痛苦	tòng-kǔ	pain and suffering	10.1
头	tóu	head	3.7
头昏	tóu-hūn	clouded head	6.7
头煎	tóu jiān	main boiling	15.5
头面	tóu-miàn	head and face	3.2
头痛	tóu-tòng	headache	3.7
头晕	tóu-yūn	dizziness	8.5
头胀	tóu-zhàng	a feeling of heaviness in the head	4.2
图	tú	plan	13.7
土	tǔ	soil	2.1
吐逆	tǔ-nì	vomit	7.4
吐痰	tǔ-tán	vomit phlegm	12.5
吐	tù	spit; vomit	4.2
吐法	tù-fǎ	the pattern of (induced) vomiting	13.2
吐血	tù-xuè	spit blood	5.7
推而至于	tuī-ér-zhì-yú	as for ...	1.4
推广	tuī-guǎng	extend	12.3
推拿	tuī-ná	manual therapy	3.8

腿	tuǐ	leg	5.5
退	tuì	push back	7.8
退却	tuì-què	abade	8.5
吞酸	tūn-suān	acid regurgitation	7.4
脱离	tuō-lí	disassociate from	3.8
唾	tuò	spittle	5.8

W

歪斜	wāi-xié	wry	3.5
外	wài	outside; external	1.4
外侧	wài-cè	outer side	1.3
外乘	wài-chéng	external affection	6.6
外感	wài-gǎn	external affection	6.6
外感病	wài-gǎn-bìng	illnesses resulting from an external affection	9.1
外感症	wài-gǎn-zhèng	pathocondition resulting from exogenous affection	11.8
外界	wài-jiè	external world; environment	5.4
外科	wài-kē	medical speciality concerned with external illnesses	1.4
外卫	wài-wèi	outer protection	4.1
外邪	wài-xié	external evil	3.5
外因	wài-yīn	external causes	6.1
顽固性	wán-gù-xìng	stubborn	12.8
顽痰	wán-tán	obstinate phlegm	13.7
丸	wán	pill	5.6
丸剂	wán-jì	pill preparations	15.1
丸药	wán-yào	pill drug	15.1

完	wán	complete; end	9.5
完备	wán-bèi	perfect; complete	14.4
完全	wán-quán	complete	8.4
完整	wán-zhěng	integrated	4.8
挽回	wǎn-huí	retrieve	13.8
挽救	wǎn-jiù	rescue	8.6
脘	wǎn	(stomach) duct	6.5
脘痞	wǎn-pǐ	blockage of the (stomach) duct	6.5
万	wàn	ten thousand	1.2
万物	wàn-wù	all things; myriad	1.2
万象	wàn-xiàng	all phenomena; myriad phenomena	1.2
亡	wáng	lose; loss	5.7
亡脱	wáng-tuō	lose; loss	5.7
亡血	wáng-xuè	blood loss	5.7
网罗	wǎng-luó	interconnect	3.1
往来	wǎng-lái	come and go; pass by	9.3
往往	wǎng-wǎng	often	4.2
旺	wàng	effulgent	5.4
望	wàng	observe; look	10.1
望诊	wàng-zhěn	visual examination	10.1
妄	wàng	erratic	5.4
妄言	wàng-yán	wild talk	10.6
微	wēi	little	6.6
危殆	wēi-dài	dangerous	8.6
危害	wēi-hài	dangerous	6.8
危急	wēi-jí	critical; in severe danger	12.7
惟	wéi	however; only	4.1
为	wéi	be; is	1.2
维持	wéi-chí	maintain	2.3
萎黄	wěi-huáng	sallow-yellow (complexion)	1.4
萎枯	wěi-kū	dry up	5.7

萎缩	wěi-suō	shrink	5.6
委靡	wěi-mǐ	tired; weak	10.1
委中	wěi-zhōng	wei-zhong (hole)	3.8
尾	wěi	tail	11.3
痿	wěi	stiff	10.4
为了	wèi-le	for; on behalf of	8.8
未	wèi	not; not yet	2.7
未 … 前	wèi … qián	before …	2.7
味	wèi	flavor (drug quality)	1.7
味	wèi	(measure word for drugs)	14.1
味道	wèi-dào	flavor	16.6
畏	wèi	fear	8.6
胃	wèi	stomach	1.5
胃病	wèi-bìng	stomach ailment	3.6
胃肠病	wèi-cháng-bìng	illness of stomach and intestines	12.8
胃腑	wèi-fǔ	the stomach	16.7
胃气	wèi-qì	stomach qi	5.1
胃热	wèi-rè	stomach heat	11.4
位置	wèi-zhì	location	1.3
谓	wèi	name; call	11.5
温	wēn	warm	1.6
温病	wēn-bìng	warmth illness	6.8
温病条辨	wēn-bìng-tiáo-biàn	(book title:) "Heat Illnesses Discussed in Individual Paragraphs"	14.4
温补	wēn-bǔ	warm supplementation	13.8
温毒症	wēn-dú-zhèng	pathocondition of warmth poisoning	13.5
温法	wēn-fǎ	(therapeutic) pattern causing a warming	1.6
温化	wēn-huà	transformation by means of warmth	13.7
温暖	wēn-nuǎn	become warm	9.4

温热	wēn-rè	warm and heat	13.1
温热药	wēn-rè-yào	warm-hot drug	16.5
温下	wēn-xià	warming purging	8.8
温性药	wēn-xìng-yào	drug of warm nature	16.5
温药	wēn-yào	warm(ing) drugs	5.8
温疫	wēn-yì	warmth epidemics	6.8
温中	wēn-zhōng	warm the center	6.3
瘟	wēn	infectious disease	6.8
瘟疫病	wēn-yì-bìng	infectious epidemic illness	10.7
文火	wén-huǒ	gentle fire	15.4
闻	wén	listen; smell	10.1
闻诊	wén-zhěn	examination by listening and smelling	10.6
紊乱	wěn-luàn	disorder	4.2
问	wèn	ask	10.8
问题	wèn-tí	issue; question	1.1
问诊	wèn-zhěn	examination by way of asking	10.8
我	wǒ	I	2.1
我们	wǒ-men	we	12.6
我们的	wǒ-men-de	our	5.2
卧	wò	lie down	6.5
屋漏	wū-lòu	leaking house (pulse condition)	11.6
无	wú	have not; do not exist	2.3
无常	wú-cháng	irregular	7.1
无从	wú cóng	have no basis from which (to do something)	12.2
无汗	wú-hàn	absence of sweating	8.2
无力	wú-lì	powerless; weak	4.3
无论	wú-lùn	regardless whether ...	3.8
无名指	wú-míng-zhǐ	ring finger	11.1
无数	wú-shù	innumerable; countless	3.4
无所谓 ...	wú suǒ wèi ...	it is impossible to speak of ...	8.5

无形	wú-xíng	formless	5.2
无以	wú-yǐ	have nothing to ...	4.2
梧桐子	wú-tóng-zǐ	wu tong seeds; seeds of Fir-miana simplex (L.) W.F. Wight	15.1
五	wǔ	five	1.3
五百	wǔ-bǎi	five hundred	15.1
五积散	wǔ-jī sǎn	powder for the five accumula-tions	14.7
五气	wǔ-qì	the five qi	6.1
五千	wǔ-qiān	five thousand	15.1
五体	wǔ-tǐ	the five (physical components constituting the) body	2.6
五味	wǔ-wèi	the five flavors	16.6
五行	wǔ-xíng	the five phases	2.1
五液	wǔ-yè	the five ye humors	5.8
五脏	wǔ-zàng	the five depots (i.e., lung, heart, spleen, liver, kidney)	1.3
五志	wǔ-zhì	the five minds	2.6
侮	wǔ	rebel; hate; humiliate	2.4
恶风	wù-fēng	aversion to wind	6.2
恶寒	wù-hán	aversion to cold	6.3
恶热	wù-rè	aversion to heat	9.2
雾	wù	fog	6.5
物	wù	item; thing; substance	4.1
物质	wù-zhì	matter; substance	1.3

X

西	xī	west	2.5
晰	xī	clear	11.5

吸	xī	inhale	6.8
吸取	xī-qǔ	absorb	15.5
吸收	xī-shōu	absorb	15.1
吸受	xī-shòu	take in through inhalation	6.8
息	xī	stop; break	3.3
息	xī	breathing	10.6
膝部	xī-bù	knee	10.5
熄	xī	calm down	13.5
犀角	xī-jiǎo	rhinoceros horn	15.2
习惯	xí-guàn	habits and customs	10.8
习惯上	xí-guàn-shàng	traditionally; usually	15.7
喜	xǐ	joy	2.6
喜欢	xǐ-huān	like; love	16.8
系	xì	belong to	1.5
系列	xì-liè	series	5.6
系统	xì-tǒng	system	4.8
细	xì	fine	8.5
细究	xì-jiū	examine closely; look (at something) closely	12.2
细小丸	xì-xiǎo-wán	very small pill	15.1
细致	xì-zhì	detailed; fine	9.1
细致地说	xì-zhì-de-shuō	strictly speaking; looked at in detail	16.5
虾游	xiā-yóu	swimming shrimp (pulse condition)	11.6
狭义	xiá-yì	narrow sense	5.5
下	xià	down; downwards; descend	1.6
下	xià	below	1.3
下	xià	apply	9.8
下达	xià-dá	defecation	13.3
下法	xià-fǎ	(therapeutic) pattern causing a downward movement; purging	1.6

下降	xià-jiàng	descend	16.3
下焦	xià-jiāo	the lower burner	1.3
下利	xià-lì	diarrhea	5.7
下消	xià-xiāo	downward wasting	5.7
夏	xià	summer	2.5
夏令	xià-lìng	summertime	6.4
夏天	xià-tiān	summer	6.8
先	xiān	first	5.3
先病	xiān-bìng	the earlier illness	12.8
先后	xiān hòu	earlier and later	12.4
先期	xiān-qī	in advance	15.1
先天	xiān-tiān	earlier dependence	4.2
咸	xián	salty	1.7
咸味	xián-wèi	salty flavor	16.6
衔接	xián-jiē	link	3.3
涎	xián	saliva	5.8
弦	xián	"string(-like)" (pulse quality)	9.3
显明	xiǎn-míng	significant	3.8
显示	xiǎn-shì	show; be a sign of	11.4
显著	xiǎn-zhù	obvious	7.2
现	xiàn	bring forth; cause to appear	1.6
现代	xiàn-dài	present	14.4
现象	xiàn-xiàng	phenomenon	1.2
现在	xiàn-zài	now	15.7
陷	xiàn	sink in	1.4
限定	xiàn-dìng	restricted	14.2
相	xiāng	mutual	1.2
相比	xiāng-bǐ	compare	5.7
相成	xiāng-chéng	be mutually complementary	1.2
相传	xiāng-chuán	transmit each other	3.2
相当	xiāng-dāng	quite	5.1

相当	xiāng-dāng	relative; certain	6.8
相得益彰	xiāng dé yì zhāng	be of mutual complementarity	14.4
相对	xiāng-duì	be mutually opposite	11.2
相反	xiāng-fǎn	be mutually opposite	1.2
相符	xiāng-fú	correspond to each other	11.8
相贯	xiāng-guàn	linked to each other	3.3
相互	xiāng-hù	mutual	2.1
相火	xiāng-huǒ	minister fire	4.5
相克	xiāng-kè	mutual restraint	2.1
相杀	xiāng-shā	relationship of killing	16.8
相生	xiāng-shēng	mutual engendering	2.1
相使	xiāng-shǐ	relationship of stimulation	16.8
相似	xiāng-sì	be similar	5.7
相随	xiāng-suí	follow each other	3.3
相提并论	xiāng-tí bìng-lùn	refer to (various things) together	4.5
相同	xiāng-tóng	be mutually identical	4.4
相畏	xiāng-wèi	relationship of awe	16.8
相侮	xiāng-wǔ	mutual rebellion	2.4
相恶	xiāng-wù	relationship of aversion	16.8
相须	xiāng-xū	relationship of accentuation	16.8
香	xiāng	aromatic; fragrant	7.5
详细	xiáng-xì	detailed	12.3
想	xiǎng	think of; consider	12.5
项	xiàng	nape	3.7
项强	xiàng-jiàng	stiff neck	8.2
向	xiàng	towards ...	9.2
象	xiàng	for example	3.7
相傅	xiàng-fù	minister	4.3
消	xiāo	dissolve	1.3
消	xiāo	waste	5.7
消除	xiāo-chú	eliminate	13.7

消导	xiāo-dǎo	digestion and transportation	12.2
消法	xiāo-fǎ	the pattern of dissolving	13.7
消化	xiāo-huà	digest; digestion	1.3
消散	xiāo-sàn	elimination through dispersion	1.8
消失	xiāo-shī	vanish	12.4
消瘦	xiāo-shòu	emaciation	1.4
消痰	xiāo-tán	dissolve phlegm	13.7
消长	xiāo-zhǎng	waning and waxing	8.1
小	xiǎo	small	11.3
小便	xiǎo-biàn	urine	4.7
小便短赤	xiǎo-biàn-duǎn-chì	short voidings of reddish urine	6.4
小便癃闭	xiǎo-biàn-lóng-bì	retention of urine	4.7
小肠	xiǎo-cháng	small intestine	4.1
小承气汤	xiǎo-chéng-qì-tāng	small decoction to contain the qi	14.5
小儿	xiǎo-ér	small children	7.5
小方	xiǎo-fāng	small formula	14.5
小溲	xiǎo-sōu	urinate; urine	8.4
小丸	xiǎo-wán	small pill	15.1
笑	xiào	laughter	4.2
效	xiào	effect	14.5
效果	xiào-guǒ	result	3.4
效能	xiào-néng	effect	14.2
效用	xiào-yòng	effect	15.1
些	xiē	some	5.2
协调	xié-tiáo	harmonize; harmony	3.4
协助	xié-zhù	support	14.2
挟	xié	in conjunction with	6.4
邪	xié	evil	3.5
邪气	xié-qì	evil qi	6.1
斜视	xié-shì	squint	10.5
胁	xié	flank	3.5

403

胁痛	xié-tòng	pain in the ribs	4.5
写	xiě	write	15.6
写方	xiě-fāng	write out a prescription	15.7
写明	xiě-míng	write out; adduce	16.1
懈怠	xiè-dài	sluggishness	4.4
泄	xiè	flow off	5.7
泄泻	xiè-xiè	diarrhea	4.3
泻	xiè	drain	1.7
泻法	xiè-fǎ	method of draining	8.8
泻下	xiè-xià	draining purgation	13.3
泻下药	xiè-xià-yào	drugs for draining downwards	13.3
泻药	xiè-yào	draining drugs	13.3
辛	xīn	acrid	1.7
辛味	xīn-wèi	acrid flavor	16.6
辛温	xīn-wēn	acrid and warming	6.3
辛夷	xīn-yí	(drug name) Magnolia liliflora Desr.	3.7
新	xīn	new; just	8.5
心	xīn	heart	2.6
心包络	xīn-bāo-luò	heart-enclosing-network	4.1
心烦	xīn-fán	vexation of the heart	6.4
心悸	xīn-jì	palpitations	4.2
心理上	xīn-lǐ-shàng	psychological	5.2
心热病	xīn-rè-bìng	heart heat illness	10.2
心神	xīn-shén	psychic constitution; mind	11.8
心脏	xīn-zàng	heart	4.1
信心	xìn-xīn	confidence	10.1
腥	xīng	rotten smell	10.7
腥臭	xīng-chòu	rotten-fetid	10.7
兴奋	xīng-fèn	exitement	1.4
形	xíng	shape	4.8
形成	xíng-chéng	form	3.4

404

形容	xíng-róng	describe	4.3
形态	xíng-tài	the condition of a person's physical appearance	10.1
形体	xíng-tǐ	the physical body	3.1
形象	xíng-xiàng	physical appearance	11.4
形状	xíng-zhuàng	shape	11.5
行	xíng	phase	2.1
行	xíng	make move; transmit	4.7
行	xíng	move	6.7
行经	xíng-jīng	menstruation	4.8
行气	xíng-qì	make qi move	5.3
行于	xíng-yú	pass through	3.2
醒	xǐng	wake up	3.5
省	xǐng	recognize; know	6.2
杏仁	xìng-rén	(drug name) Prunus armeniaca L.	14.3
性	xìng	nature	1.4
性能	xìng-néng	ability; effect	16.4
性欲	xìng-yù	libido	4.4
性质	xìng-zhì	quality; nature	1.3
胸	xiōng	chest	5.3
胸闷	xiōng-mèn	chest pressure	4.5
胸中有	xiōng-zhōng yǒu	have in mind	15.7
熊胆	xióng-dǎn	bear's gall	15.2
修	xiū	study; care about	3.1
修治	xiū-zhì	trim and manage (general designation of the pharmaceutical processing of Chinese drugs)	16.2
嗅觉	xiù-jué	sense of smelling	10.6
需要	xū-yào	must; needs to	5.3
虚	xū	depletion	1.8
虚	xū	depleted (pulse condition)	11.2

虚寒	xū-hán	depletion cold	11.4
虚寒症	xū-hán-zhèng	pathoconditions of depletion cold	9.4
虚热	xū-rè	depletion heat	13.5
虚弱	xū-ruò	depleted and weak	5.8
虚脱	xū-tuō	loss	13.8
虚症	xū-zhèng	pathocondition of depletion	4.3
须	xū	must	5.4
须臾	xū-yú	moment	11.6
许多	xǔ-duō	many	8.7
叙	xù	assess	15.6
叙述	xù-shù	discuss; outline	8.1
序	xù	order	11.6
宣	xuān	disperse	14.3
宣肺法	xuān-fèi-fǎ	pattern of transmitting the lung (qi)	13.1
宣通	xuān-tōng	promote an unimpeded flow	13.1
选择	xuǎn-zé	select	13.1
削	xuē	cut	12.3
学术	xué-shù	science	14.4
学说	xué-shuō	theory; doctrine	1.1
学习	xué-xí	study	9.8
穴	xué	hole; opening	3.6
血	xuè	blood	1.3
血病	xuè-bìng	blood illness	5.4
血分	xuè-fèn	blood section	13.5
血分病	xuè-fèn-bìng	illnesses in the section of the blood; blood illnesses	5.3
血分热	xuè-fèn-rè	heat in the blood section	13.5
血分药	xuè-fèn-yào	drugs active in the section of the blood	5.3
血寒	xuè-hán	blood cold	1.5

血竭	xuè-jié	(drug name) Daemonorops draco Bl.; dragon's blood	15.2
血亏	xuè-kuī	anemia	5.4
血热	xuè-rè	blood heat	1.5
血少	xuè-shǎo	diminished blood	11.4
血脱	xuè-tuō	blood loss	5.3
血虚	xuè-xū	blood depletion	1.5
血液	xuè-yè	blood	1.5
血症	xuè-zhèng	blood condition	7.8
循	xún	follow; along with	3.3
循环不息	xún huán bù xī	circular flow without pause	3.3
循经传	xún-jīng-chuán	transmission following the conduits	9.6
循行	xún-xíng	penetrate; pass through	3.2
循衣	xún-yī	follow the clothes (with the hands)	10.5
寻	xún	search	11.8
寻求	xún-qiú	investigate	11.1
迅速	xùn-sù	speedy	12.6

Y

焉	yān	(final particle)	11.5
咽干	yān-gān	dry throat	6.6
咽喉	yān-hóu	throat	6.6
咽痛	yān-tòng	pharyngeal pain	9.4
盐水制	yán-shuǐ-zhì	processing with brine	16.3
盐水	yán-shuǐ	brine	16.3
严重	yán-zhòng	serious	5.3

研	yán	grind	15.1
研成	yán-chéng	grind into ...	15.1
研究	yán-jiū	research	3.4
言	yán	speak; refer to	4.4
言语	yán-yǔ	speech	4.3
颜	yán	forehead	10.2
颜色	yán-sè	color	10.4
沿用	yán-yòng	remain in use	16.3
眼	yǎn	eye	3.5
眼眶	yǎn-kuàng	eye socket	7.5
演绎	yǎn-yì	deduct	8.1
阳病	yáng-bìng	yang illness	1.6
阳经	yáng-jīng	yang conduits	3.2
阳脉	yáng-mài	yang pulse	1.5
阳明	yáng-míng	yang brilliance	9.1
阳明病	yáng-míng-bìng	yang brilliance illness	9.2
阳明腑	yáng-míng-fǔ	yang brilliance palace	9.2
阳明经	yáng-míng-jīng	yang brilliance conduit	3.7
阳明脉	yáng-míng-mài	yang brilliance vessel	9.2
阳气	yáng-qì	yang qi	5.1
阳盛	yáng-shèng	yang abundance	1.4
阳胜	yáng-shèng	yang domination	1.6
阳虚	yáng-xū	yang depletion	1.4
阳虚症	yáng-xū-zhèng	pathocondition of yang depletion	13.8
阳药	yáng-yào	yang drug	1.7
阳症	yáng-zhèng	yang pathocondition	1.4
养	yǎng	nourish	4.8
养血	yǎng-xuè	nourish the blood	5.6
样	yàng	type	10.7
要求	yāo-qiú	requirement	15.1
腰	yāo	lumbus	5.6

腰酸	yāo-suān	lumbar pain	5.5
腰痛	yāo-tòng	lumbago	4.4
摇	yáo	tremble	11.5
咬伤	yǎo-shāng	injury from a bite	7.7
窅	yǎo	indentation	11.7
杳	yǎo	vanish without traces	11.6
药	yào	drug	1.7
药方	yào-fāng	formula; prescription	7.8
药粉	yào-fěn	drug powder	15.2
药酒	yào-jiǔ	medicinal wine	15.4
药理	yào-lǐ	principles of drug (effects)	16.4
药理作用	yào-lǐ-zuò-yòng	pharmacological effect	16.4
药力	yào-lì	drug force	14.3
药量	yào-liàng	quantity of drugs	14.6
药丸	yào-wán	drug pill	15.1
药味	yào-wèi	medicinal drug	15.7
药物	yào-wù	pharmaceutics; medical drugs	1.1
药物性能	yào-wù-xìng-néng	drug ability	16.2
药物中毒	yào-wù-zhòng-dú	drug poisoning	7.7
药性	yào-xìng	drug quality	1.7
药汁	yào-zhī	drug extract	15.5
要	yào	wish	1.8
要	yào	certainly; definitely	15.7
噎膈	yē-gé	esophageal constriction	6.6
也	yě	too; also	1.3
也就是	yě-jiù-shì	in other words	2.2
叶天士	yè tiān-shì	(author's name) Ye Tianshi	15.8
夜	yè	night	1.2
液	yè	liquid	1.5
液质	yè-zhì	humors	5.7
一	yī	one	1.1

一	yī	as soon as	9.6
一般	yī-bān	in general; generally	1.4
一般的说	yī-bān-de-shuō	generally speaking	1.3
一定	yī-dìng	definite; specific	2.5
一行一行	yī-háng-yī-háng	column after column	15.7
一排一排	yī-pái-yī-pái	line after line	15.7
一千	yī-qiān	one thousand	15.1
一切	yī-qiè	all; each	1.2
一万	yī-wàn	ten thousand	15.1
一些	yī-xiē	some	3.7
一样	yī-yàng	in the same way	2.7
一致	yī-zhì	identical	4.1
医	yī	medicine	1.1
医案	yī-àn	medical case histories	15.8
医疗	yī-liáo	treat; therapy	1.1
医生	yī-shēng	physician	10.1
医学	yī-xué	medicine	1.1
医者	yī-zhě	physicians	3.1
依	yī	depend on	2.5
依 ... 来	yī ... lái	in accordance with	2.5
依次	yī-cì	in succession; in proper order; one after another	15.7
依据	yī-jù	foundation	3.6
衣	yī	clothing	6.5
遗	yí	lose	1.4
遗	yí	uncontrolled flow	3.5
遗精	yí-jīng	seminal emission	1.4
遗溺	yí-niào	enuresis	4.7
移	yí	move	6.2
移时	yí-shí	in the course of time	6.2
疑	yí	doubt	7.1
宜	yí	should; appropriate	2.7

已	yǐ	already	2.7
已 ... 时 , 则 ...	yǐ ... shí, zé ...	if already ..., then ...	2.7
已经	yǐ-jīng	already	3.8
已往	yǐ-wǎng	earlier; in the past	10.8
乙	yǐ	second (in an enumeration)	2.8
... 以后	... yǐ-hòu	after ...	5.5
以	yǐ	in order to; for	1.2
以	yǐ	take; by means of	1.3
以 ... 来说	yǐ ... lái shuō	as far as ... is concerned	1.5
以 ... 为例	yǐ ... wéi lì	take ... as an example	2.1
以 ... 为主	yǐ ... wéi-zhǔ	rest mainly on ...	3.4
以 A 为 B	yǐ A wéi B	consider A as B	1.3
以便	yǐ-biàn	in order to	2.6
以及	yǐ-jí	as well as; up to	2.5
以偏救偏	yǐ-piān-jiù-piān	save the unilateral with the unilateral	16.4
以前	yǐ-qián	before; in the past	14.4
以上	yǐ-shàng	above	3.7
抑郁	yì-yù	depression	7.1
易	yì	easy	4.3
易怒	yì-nù	tendency to become angry	4.5
逸	yì	idleness	5.2
疫疠	yì-lì	epidemics	6.8
亦	yì	still	8.6
亦	yì	also	2.4
意乱	yì-luàn	mental chaos	7.1
意思	yì-si	meaning	4.2
意外	yì-wài	accident	7.7
意义	yì-yì	meaning; significance	1.6
益	yì	increase	5.3
益火	yì-huǒ	boost fire	2.8
益精	yì-jīng	increase the semen	13.8

益气	yì-qì	increase qi	5.3
异	yì	be different	5.1
异常	yì-cháng	abnormal	7.5
异乎寻常	yì-hū-xún-cháng	unusual	4.8
因	yīn	follow; because	4.2
因此	yīn-cǐ	hence	1.8
因而	yīn-ér	hence	1.4
因素	yīn-sù	element; factor	5.2
因为	yīn-wèi	because	5.3
因阵	yīn-zhèn	adapted array	14.7
音嘎	yīn-gā	hoarse voice	13.1
音哑	yīn-yǎ	loss of voice	16.2
阴病	yīn-bìng	yin illness	1.6
阴分	yīn-fèn	yin section	10.4
阴经	yīn-jīng	yin conduits	3.2
阴脉	yīn-mài	yin pulse	1.5
阴盛	yīn-shèng	yin abundance	1.4
阴胜	yīn-shèng	yin domination	1.6
阴邪	yīn-xié	yin evil	6.3
阴虚	yīn-xū	yin depletion	1.4
阴虚症	yīn-xū-zhèng	pathocondition of yin depletion	13.8
阴阳	yīn yáng	yin and yang (the two principles and basic categories of all being)	1.1
阴药	yīn-yào	yin drug	1.7
阴症	yīn-zhèng	yin pathocondition	1.4
银花	yín-huā	(drug name) Lonicera japonica Thunb. L.	1.7
淫雨	yín-yǔ	excessive rain	6.8
龈	yín	gums	3.6
龈肿	yín-zhǒng	swollen gums	3.6
饮	yǐn	drink	5.8

饮食	yǐn-shí	drink and food	5.4
引	yǐn	draw	8.6
引长	yǐn-cháng	protract	10.6
引到	yǐn-dào	guide	14.3
引发	yǐn-fā	bring forth	7.6
引经药	yǐn-jīng-yào	conduit guiding drug	14.3
引起	yǐn-qǐ	cause; set off	1.8
引药	yǐn-yào	guiding drug	14.3
引用	yǐn-yòng	apply; make use of	9.1
应	yīng	should, must	1.8
应	yīng	respond (to the pressure of a finger)	11.2
应当	yīng-dāng	should; must	2.7
应该	yīng-gāi	should, must	1.8
营	yíng	nourish	3.1
营	yíng	blood; constructive (qi)	13.5
营养	yíng-yǎng	nourishment	4.3
迎刃而解	yíng-rèn-ér-jiě	solve easily	12.5
影响	yǐng-xiǎng	influence	3.8
瘿瘤	yǐng-liú	goiter	7.3
硬	yìng	hard	10.4
应用	yìng-yòng	apply	1.8
壅塞	yōng-sè	blockage	13.2
壅滞	yōng-zhì	obstruction	13.7
涌	yǒng	gush forth; well up	11.6
涌吐	yǒng-tù	ejection through vomiting	13.2
勇敢	yǒng-gǎn	courage	4.5
用	yòng	with ... (+ verb)	15.7
用	yòng	employ; use	1.1
用 ... 来	yòng ... lái	with	1.3
用 ... 作	yòng ... zuò ...	use .. for ...	15.4
用处	yòng-chu	application	12.2

用法	yòng-fǎ	application	8.8
用药	yòng-yào	drug use	1.7
忧	yōu	anxiety	2.6
忧虑	yōu-lǜ	worry	10.1
尤	yóu	especially	7.5
尤其是	yóu-qí-shì	especially	13.5
尤在泾	yóu zài-jīng	(author's name:) You Zaijing	9.8
由	yóu	from; take its origin in	3.3
由于	yóu-yú	because of ...	3.3
油	yóu	oil; oily	7.4
有	yǒu	some	16.7
有	yǒu	have; exist	1.2
有的	yǒu-de	some	7.5
有关	yǒu-guān	be related to	4.8
有机	yǒu-jī	organic	3.3
有利	yǒu-lì	beneficial	10.1
有力	yǒu-lì	have strength; strong	11.2
有时	yǒu-shí	sometimes; occasionally	2.4
有所	yǒu suǒ	there is something which; a little	12.3
有无	yǒu-wú	whether or not	5.8
有限	yǒu-xiàn	limited	15.8
有效	yǒu-xiào	effective	5.3
有些	yǒu-xiē	there are some; some	5.2
有形	yǒu-xíng	tangible	5.2
有余	yǒu-yú	be present in surplus	2.4
右	yòu	right	3.3
右尺	yòu-chǐ	right foot	11.1
右寸	yòu-cùn	right inch	11.1
右关	yòu-guān	right gate	11.1
又	yòu	still; again	1.2

414

又如	yòu-rú	as a further example; on the other hand	7.8
幼	yòu	child; youth	3.8
瘀	yū	stagnate; stagnation	5.3
瘀血	yū-xuè	stagnant blood	5.3
于	yú	at; in	1.2
于此可见	yú-cǐ-kě-jiàn	that shows; from this it can be seen	12.3
余	yú	surplus	2.4
余气	yú-qì	residual qi	6.6
鱼翔	yú-xiáng	waving fish (pulse condition)	11.6
予	yǔ	give	12.2
与	yǔ	and; with	2.1
与...相	yǔ ... xiāng	in comparison with	4.1
与...相同	yǔ ... xiāng-tóng	identical with ...; correspond to each other	4.4
与否	yǔ-fǒu	or not	9.5
宇宙	yǔ-zhòu	universe	1.2
语	yǔ	language; speech	10.6
语气	yǔ-qì	intonation	10.6
语言	yǔ-yán	speech	6.2
玉竹	yù-zhú	(drug name) Polygonatum odoratum (Mill.) Druce and other Polygonatum species	5.8
郁	yù	depressed; impeded	2.7
郁火	yù-huǒ	depressed fire	13.2
郁蒸	yù-zhēng	heavy steaming	6.4
遇到	yù-dào	encounter	3.5
愈	yù	even more	6.4
欲	yù	wish	5.8
欲寐	yù-mèi	desire to sleep	9.4
预后	yù-hòu	prognosis	10.1
预为	yù-wéi	prepare	2.7

元气	yuán-qì	original qi	5.1
原是	yuán-shì	is/are basically	12.7
原因	yuán-yīn	cause	7.8
原则	yuán-zé	guiding principle	12.8
圆形体	yuán-xíng-tǐ	round-shaped body	15.1
源	yuán	source	5.7
约制	yuē-zhì	restrict	2.2
越	yuè	skip; bypass	9.6
越出	yuè-chū	transgress; leave	6.1
越经传	yuè-jīng-chuán	transmission bypassing (one or two) conduits	9.6
月	yuè	moon	1.2
月经	yuè-jīng	monthly period; menstruation	13.4
阅读	yuè-dú	read	9.8
云茯苓	yún-fú-líng	(the drug) fuling from (the province of) Yun(nan)	16.1
匀	yún	even	11.3
运	yùn	transport	4.3
运化	yùn-huà	movement and transformation; digestion	7.4
运输	yùn-shū	transport	4.3
运行	yùn-xíng	transmission	3.3
运用	yùn-yòng	apply	1.8
酝酿	yùn-niàng	ferment	6.8

Z

杂	zá	various; mixed	7.5
杂病	zá-bìng	miscellaneous illnesses	13.4

416

哉	zāi	(particle emphasizing the preceding statement)	11.5
再	zài	again	2.2
再次	zài-cì	still another	13.7
在	zài	be there; exist	16.7
在	zài	in; at	1.1
在	zài	(particle indicating the continuous form of the subsequent verb)	5.6
在 ... 的	zài ... de	being in ...	3.1
在 ... 方面	zài ... fāng-miàn	as for ...	1.3
在 ... 上	zài ... shàng	in ...; as for ...	1.3
在 ... 时	zài ... shí	while; during ...	2.8
在 ... 时候	zài ... shí-hòu	while; during ...	5.6
在 ... 下	zài ... xià	under ...	2.4
在 ... 中	zài ... zhōng	within ...	2.4
在 ... 中的	zài ... zhōng de	being present in ...	1.1
在于	zài-yú	be in; take place in	16.7
脏病	zàng-bìng	illnesses of the depots	2.8
脏腑	zàng-fǔ	the inner organs	1.3
脏器	zàng-qì	depot organ	3.8
脏气	zàng-qì	qi in the depots	10.3
糟	zāo	residues of fermentation	11.7
糟粕	zāo-pò	waste	4.6
早	zǎo	early	14.4
早泄	zǎo-xiè	premature ejaculation	4.4
造成	zào-chéng	bring forth	7.8
燥	zào	parched	1.5
燥裂	zào-liè	dry out and crack	6.6
燥屎	zào-shǐ	dry faeces	9.2
燥痰	zào-tán	dryness-phlegm	7.3
燥症	zào-zhèng	dryness pathoconditions	6.6

则	zé	then	1.6
增加	zēng-jiā	increase	8.6
渣滓	zhā-zǐ	solid dregs	4.6
沾	zhān	wet	6.5
谵语	zhān-yǔ	wild talk	4.2
占	zhàn	assume (a stage)	12.7
占有	zhàn-yǒu	have	7.3
战	zhàn	mobile	10.4
战胜	zhàn-shèng	be victorious	12.1
战术	zhàn-shù	tactics	12.3
战术上	zhàn-shù shàng	in tactics	12.3
樟脑	zhāng-nǎo	camphor	15.2
章	zhāng	chapter	8.1
章	zhāng	display	10.8
张景岳	zhāng jǐng-yuè	(author's name:) Zhang Jingyue	10.8
张力	zhāng-lì	tension	3.8
张仲景	zhāng zhòng-jǐng	(author's name) Zhang Zhong-jing	14.4
长	zhǎng	chief	6.2
长	zhǎng	grow; growth	2.5
掌	zhǎng	palm	11.1
掌握	zhǎng-wò	grasp	8.1
胀	zhàng	distension	4.2
胀满	zhàng-mǎn	swelling and fullness	4.7
胀痛	zhàng-tòng	pressure and pain	6.7
障碍	zhàng-ài	obstruction	5.3
招致	zhāo-zhì	invite	7.7
着	zháo	reach; get to; press against	11.2
找到	zhǎo-dào	find out	8.1
找寻	zhǎo-xún	search	12.5
折	zhé	break	6.7

者	zhě	(particle defining the immediately preceding verb or number as a noun referring to an item or to a person; here: wu zhe "the five"; zhe wu zhe "these five")	2.1
这	zhè	this; these	1.2
这就	zhè-jiù	that is	5.6
这类	zhè-lèi	such	9.7
这里	zhè-lǐ	here	8.4
这些	zhè-xiē	these	2.8
这样	zhè-yàng	such	2.1
这一	zhè-yī	this	2.6
这种	zhè-zhǒng	this	9.5
浙贝母	zhè-bèi-mǔ	(the drug) beimu from (the province of Zhe)jiang	16.1
浙江	zhè-jiāng	(name of province) Zhejiang	16.1
着	zhe	(particle defining the immediately preceding verb as a gerund; roughly equivalent to the English "..ing")	1.1
珍珠	zhēn-zhū	pearl	15.2
真	zhēn	true	3.5
真气	zhēn-qì	true qi	5.1
真相	zhēn-xiàng	the real facts	8.7
真阳	zhēn-yáng	true yang (qi)	5.1
真阴	zhēn-yīn	true yin (qi)	5.1
真正	zhēn-zhèng	true; indeed; really	12.2
针	zhēn	needle	3.6
针刺	zhēn-cì	needling	3.6
针对	zhēn-duì	focus on	12.1
针灸	zhēn-jiǔ	acupuncture and moxa therapy	3.8
诊	zhěn	examine; diagnose	1.5

诊断	zhěn-duàn	diagnosis	1.1
振掉	zhèn-diào	sway	10.5
镇	zhèn	press down	13.5
镇静	zhèn-jìng	tranquilize	13.5
阵痛	zhèn-tòng	the pains of birth	7.5
蒸	zhēng	steam	16.2
蒸制	zhēng-zhì	process by steaming	16.2
征象	zhēng-xiàng	sign	8.1
整个	zhěng-gè	entire	4.6
整套	zhěng-tào	complete system; set	1.1
整体	zhěng-tǐ	whole	3.3
正	zhèng	proper; regular; normal	1.2
正常	zhèng-cháng	normal	4.2
正反	zhèng-fǎn	norm and opposite	1.2
正骨	zhèng-gǔ	chiropractice; bone correcting	3.8
正面	zhèng-miàn	front side; frontal	12.1
正气	zhèng-qì	proper qi	6.1
正在	zhèng-zài	be just (in a specific state)	13.4
正治	zhèng-zhì	direct treatment	12.1
正治法	zhèng-zhì-fǎ	pattern of a direct therapy	12.2
症	zhèng	pathocondition	1.4
症候	zhèng-hòu	symptoms	2.7
症象	zhèng-xiàng	sign	8.6
症状	zhèng-zhuàng	pathomanifestation	1.4
证	zhèng	evidence; sign; (illness) manifestations	9.8
证明	zhèng-míng	demonstrate	3.8
证实	zhèng-shí	evidence	3.8
癥瘕	zhèng-jiǎ	concretion	13.7
支	zhī	(measure word for conduits, branches, and sidelines)	3.2

知母	zhī-mǔ	(drug name) Anemarrhena asphodeloides Bge.	16.5
知识	zhī-shí	knowledge	15.6
肢	zhī	limb; extremity	3.2
肢冷	zhī-lěng	cold limbs	6.3
肢末	zhī-mò	the ends of the limbs	3.2
肢软	zhī-ruǎn	soft limbs	6.4
汁	zhī	juice; extract	15.3
之	zhī	this	12.3
之	zhī	(particle identifying the immediately preceding expression as a possessive)	2.1
之后	zhī-hòu	following; after	6.6
之间	zhī-jiān	among; between	2.3
之外	zhī-wài	in addition to	4.8
之一	zhī-yī	one of ...	3.4
职司	zhí-sī	regulate; manage	4.6
直	zhí	straight; lengthwise	3.1
直	zhí	direct	6.7
直接	zhí-jiē	direct	2.6
直中	zhí-zhòng	direct strike	9.6
植物	zhí-wù	plant	16.1
植物油	zhí-wù-yóu	vegetable oil	15.3
执	zhí	cling to	10.2
值得	zhí-de	be worth	3.8
指	zhǐ	finger	11.1
指	zhǐ	refer to	1.8
指...而言	zhǐ ... ér yán	refer to	4.4
指出	zhǐ-chū	point out	16.7
指导	zhǐ-dǎo	guide	1.1
指示	zhǐ-shì	refer to	8.1
止	zhǐ	stop	11.3

止血	zhǐ-xuè	stop bleeding	12.5
只	zhǐ	only	7.2
只是	zhǐ-shì	it is just that	15.6
只要	zhǐ-yào	all that is necessary is	13.2
只有	zhǐ-yǒu	only if	1.8
纸	zhǐ	paper	15.3
至	zhì	arrive; reach	1.5
至 ... 为度	zhì ... wéi dù	until ...	15.3
至 ... 为止	zhì ... wéi zhǐ	until ...	15.2
至数	zhì-shù	pulse frequency (arrival of pulses)	1.5
至于	zhì-yú	as for; as far as	12.3
致病	zhì-bìng	lead to illness	7.4
致病因素	zhì-bìng-yīn-sù	factors leading to illness	6.1
置	zhì	bring; put	15.2
制	zhì	scope	14.5
制	zhì	control; check; process	16.2
制成	zhì-chéng	prepare	15.1
制法	zhì-fǎ	production method	15.3
制过	zhì-guò	control drawbacks	16.2
制化	zhì-huà	construction and counterreaction	2.3
滞	zhì	sluggish	5.3
治	zhì	treat	2.7
治本	zhì-běn	treat the root (of an illness)	12.7
治标	zhì-biāo	treat the tip (of an illness)	12.7
治法	zhì-fǎ	therapeutic pattern	2.8
治疗	zhì-liáo	treat; therapy	1.1
中	zhōng	in; amidst	1.1
中	zhōng	Chinese	1.1
中间	zhōng-jiān	be between	9.3
中焦	zhōng-jiāo	central burner	4.7

中气	zhōng-qì	central qi	5.1
中西医	zhōng-xī-yī	Chinese and Western medicine	3.8
中心	zhōng-xīn	center	10.3
中虚（症）	zhōng-xū-(zhèng)	(pathocondition of) central depletion	13.5
中药	zhōng-yào	traditional Chinese drug	1.7
中药方	zhōng-yào-fāng	prescription of Chinese drugs; Chinese pharmaceutical prescriptions	15.7
中药学	zhōng-yào-xué	Chinese pharmaceutics	3.6
中医学	zhōng-yī-xué	Chinese medicine	1.1
中医	zhōng yī	Chinese medicine	1.1
中指	zhōng-zhǐ	middle finger	11.1
终	zhōng	end	9.6
终身	zhōng-shēn	the entire life	15.8
种	zhǒng	type; (measure word for abstract concepts)	1.2
种类	zhǒng-lèi	kind; type	14.5
肿	zhǒng	swell; swelling	1.4
肿疡	zhǒng-yáng	lesion	1.8
种子	zhòng-zǐ	fertility	4.2
中	zhòng	strike	3.5
中毒	zhòng-dú	poisoning	7.7
中风	zhòng-fēng	struck by wind	3.5
中寒	zhòng-hán	cold stroke	6.3
中暑	zhòng-shǔ	summerheat stroke	6.4
中暍	zhòng-yè	sunstroke	6.4
重	zhòng	heavy; serious	3.5
重按	zhòng-àn	press heavily	11.1
重大	zhòng-dà	important	3.1
重量	zhòng-liàng	weight	15.1
重视	zhòng-shì	regard highly; pay attention to	2.8

重要	zhòng-yào	important	3.1
重要性	zhòng-yào-xìng	importance	3.8
重症	zhòng-zhèng	serious pathocondition	10.2
众	zhòng	numerous	14.4
州都	zhōu-dū	"Regional Rectifier" (ancient offical title)	4.7
肘	zhǒu	ellbow	3.5
昼	zhòu	daytime	1.2
骤	zhòu	dramatically; suddenly	8.6
朱砂	zhū-shā	cinnabar	5.6
猪腰	zhū-yāo	pig's kidneys	10.4
诸	zhū	all	11.4
潴汇	zhū-huì	gather water	4.7
逐	zhú	follow	3.2
逐	zhú	eliminate; expel	5.3
逐寒	zhú-hán	eliminate cold	13.6
逐渐	zhú-jiàn	slowly; gradually	13.6
逐经	zhú-jīng	one conduit after another	3.2
逐瘀	zhú-yū	expel stagnations	5.3
主	zhǔ	master; be responsible for	1.3
主	zhǔ	rule; indicate	10.2
主持	zhǔ-chí	direct; be responsible for	5.6
主脉	zhǔ-mài	main pulses	9.7
主气	zhǔ-qì	ruling qi	6.4
主司	zhǔ-sī	be responsible for	1.3
主要	zhǔ-yào	basically; in principle	1.6
主药	zhǔ-yào	master drug	3.7
主因	zhǔ-yīn	major cause	7.6
主宰	zhǔ-zǎi	ruler	4.2
主症	zhǔ-zhèng	main pathoconditions	9.7
著作	zhù-zuò	writing	14.4
助药	zhù-yào	supporting drug	15.7

助长	zhù-zhǎng	support	2.1
贮藏	zhù-cáng	store	4.1
注	zhù	comment	9.8
注解	zhù-jiě	comment	9.8
注意	zhù-yì	pay attention	3.8
抓住	zhuā-zhù	get a hold of	12.5
专	zhuān	only; exclusively	7.8
专门	zhuān-mén	exclusively; specialized	3.8
专一	zhuān-yī	concentrated	14.6
转变	zhuǎn-biàn	transformation	10.8
转侧	zhuǎn-cè	turn to the side	5.6
转化	zhuǎn-huà	transform	5.7
转输	zhuǎn-shū	forward; transfer; pass along	4.1
转索	zhuǎn-suǒ	twisted rope	11.3
转为	zhuǎn-wéi	change into	8.6
转	zhuàn	turn around	5.6
撰述	zhuàn-shù	compile	14.4
妆	zhuāng	make-up; rouge	7.5
壮	zhuàng	strong	8.5
壮热	zhuàng-rè	strong heat	6.4
状	zhuàng	appearance	11.6
准确	zhǔn-què	real; realistic	10.2
准则	zhǔn-zé	criterion	3.4
着手	zhuó-shǒu	treat	4.6
着重	zhuó-zhòng	emphasize	3.2
浊	zhuó	turbid	4.6
兹	zī	here; now	8.1
资生	zī-shēng	create	2.1
姿态	zī-tài	posture	10.5
滋补	zī-bǔ	nourish and supplement	13.1
滋润法	zī-rùn-fǎ	moistening (therapy) pattern	12.2

滋肾	zī-shèn	enrich the kidneys	2.7
滋养	zī-yǎng	nourish	1.7
仔细	zǐ-xì	carefully	7.2
子	zǐ	son	2.1
子宫	zǐ-gōng	uterus	3.8
自	zì	from	3.3
自	zì	self	4.2
自	zì	of course	12.5
自	zì	self; automatic; spontaneous	5.8
自汗	zì-hàn	spontaneous sweating	6.4
自己	zì-jǐ	self; own	15.8
自觉	zì-jué	subjective	10.8
自利	zì-lì	spontaneous discharges	9.3
自然	zì-rán	nature; natural	1.2
自然界	zì-rán-jiè	the natural world; nature	2.5
自上而下	zì shàng ér xià	from above downwards	3.3
自主	zì-zhǔ	self-control	4.2
自主力	zì-zhǔ-lì	power of self-determination	10.1
字	zì	character of Chinese script	5.3
恣	zì	unrestrained	7.4
宗气	zōng-qì	ancestral qi	5.1
综合	zōng-hé	comprehensive	14.1
总	zǒng	always	4.1
总按	zǒng-àn	feel (with all three fingers) together	11.1
总的说来	zǒng-de-shuō-lái	generally speaking	7.1
总括	zǒng-kuò	survey	11.5
总之	zǒng-zhī	in general; to sum up	13.8
走	zǒu	go; move	3.3
足	zú	sufficient	4.7
足	zú	foot	11.7
足三里	zú-sān-lǐ	the leg san-li (hole)	3.6

阻	zǔ	blocked	3.5
阻碍	zǔ-ài	block	7.3
组成	zǔ-chéng	constitute; constitutive	3.1
组成部分	zǔ-chéng bù-fèn	constitutive element	3.1
组织	zǔ-zhī	structure; tissue; organization	2.5
最	zuì	very; extreme	4.3
最后	zuì-hòu	very last	4.6
最为	zuì-wéi	be most... (to express superlative)	6.7
最早	zuì-zǎo	earliest	9.1
尊为	zūn-wéi	revere as	14.4
左	zuǒ	left	3.3
左尺	zuǒ-chǐ	left foot	11.1
左寸	zuǒ-cùn	left inch	11.1
左关	zuǒ-guān	left gate	11.1
左瘫右痪	zuǒ-tān-yòu-huàn	left and right side paralysis	3.5
佐	zuǒ	assist	2.7
佐药	zuǒ-yào	assistant drug	14.3
作	zuò	make	4.3
作	zuò	serve as	11.1
作成	zuò-chéng	form to ...	15.1
作出	zuò-chū	produce; generate	9.1
作痛	zuò-tòng	cause pain	11.7
作为	zuò-wéi	consider as ...	3.4
作痒	zuò-yǎng	itch	7.5
作业	zuò-yè	work	6.5
作用	zuò-yòng	function; effect	1.3
坐	zuò	sit	6.5

Further titles on Chinese medicine by Paul U.Unschuld:

1. Philology

Introductory Readings in Classical Chinese Medicine.
Sixty Texts with Vocabulary and Translation, a Guide to Research Aids
and a General Glossary, 463 pp.
Kluwer Academic Publishers. Dordrecht, Boston, London.

Approaches to Ancient Chinese Medical Literature.
Proceedings of an International Symposium on Translation
Methodologies and Terminologies. 175 pp.
Kluwer Academic Publishers. Dordrecht, Boston, London.

2. Text editions

Nan-ching. The Classic of Difficult Issues.
An annotated translation of this first century classic with commentaries
by 20 Chinese and Japanese authors from the 3rd to the 19th century,
and the original text in Chinese. 760 pp.
University of California Press. Berkeley, Los Angeles, London.

Forgotten Traditions of Ancient Chinese Medicine.
A Chinese View from the Eighteenth Century.
An annotated translation of the *Yi xue yuan liu lun* by Xu Dachun of
1757 with the original text in Chinese. 403 pp.
Paradigm Publishing Co.. Brookline/Ma. USA

with J.Kovacs: **Subtleties on the Silver Sea.**
An annotated translation of the ophthalmological classic *Yin-hai jing-
wei* of about the 15th century with the original text in Chinese. 460 pp.
University of California Press. Berkeley, Los Angeles, London.

3. General studies

Medicine in China. A History of Pharmaceutics. 366 pp.
University of California Press. Berkeley, Los Angeles, London.

Medicine in China. A History of Ideas. 423 pp.
University of California Press. Berkeley, Los Angeles, London.

A set of two cassettes as a pronunciation aid for **Learn To Read
Chinese** is available. The tapes provide the texts of lessons one
through sixteen as read by a native Chinese speaker